ATKINS DIET COOKBOOK FOR BEGINNERS 2024

Atkins Diet Made Easy: Flavorful Recipes for Weight Loss,healthy living and a Low-Carb Lifestyle

By

DR.Ashley McGrane

Table of contents

Chapter 1: Introduction to the Atkins Diet

The Atkins Diet, developed by Dr. Robert Atkins in the 1960s, is a low-carbohydrate eating plan designed to promote weight loss and improve overall health. It focuses on limiting carbohydrate intake while encouraging the consumption of protein and healthy fats. This dietary approach aims to shift the body's metabolism from burning carbohydrates for energy to burning stored fat, leading to rapid weight loss and potentially other health benefits. Throughout its evolution, the Atkins Diet has gained popularity and undergone modifications, offering various phases and options to suit individual preferences and goals.

The Atkins Diet is divided into several phases, typically starting with a strict restriction of carbohydrates, followed by a gradual reintroduction of carbohydrates as weight loss goals are achieved. Here's an overview of the key phases:

1. Induction Phase: This initial phase lasts about two weeks and involves severely limiting carbohydrate intake to around 20-25 grams per day. During this phase, the body enters a state of ketosis, where it burns fat for fuel instead of carbohydrates. Foods allowed during this phase include protein sources like meat, fish, eggs, and certain cheeses, as well as non-starchy vegetables and fats like butter and olive oil.

2. Ongoing Weight Loss (OWL) Phase: In this phase, carbohydrates are gradually reintroduced into the diet in small increments, typically around 5 grams per week. This phase continues until the individual is within 10 pounds of their target weight. More variety in food choices is introduced during this phase, including nuts, seeds, berries, and low-carb vegetables.

3. Pre-Maintenance Phase: Once close to the target weight, individuals move to the Pre-Maintenance Phase, where carbohydrate intake is increased slightly to find the level that allows weight maintenance without gaining or losing. This phase helps individuals identify their personal carbohydrate tolerance level.

4. Maintenance Phase: In the Maintenance Phase, individuals have reached their target weight and continue to follow the principles of the Atkins Diet to maintain their weight loss and overall health. This phase emphasizes a balanced approach to eating, focusing on whole foods, adequate protein, healthy fats, and controlled carbohydrates.

Understanding the principles of the Atkins Diet

The Atkins Diet is based on several core principles aimed at promoting weight loss and improving overall health. Here are the fundamental principles of the Atkins Diet:

1. Limit Carbohydrate Intake: The Atkins Diet emphasizes reducing carbohydrate intake, especially simple carbohydrates like sugars and refined grains. By restricting carbohydrates, the body is forced to burn stored fat for fuel, leading to weight loss.

2. Focus on Protein and Healthy Fats: While carbohydrates are limited, the diet encourages the consumption of protein and healthy fats. Protein helps maintain muscle mass and promotes satiety, while healthy fats provide essential nutrients and help keep you feeling full.

3. Phased Approach: The Atkins Diet is divided into phases to gradually reintroduce carbohydrates while monitoring weight loss progress. This phased approach helps individuals find their optimal carbohydrate intake for weight loss and maintenance.

4. Emphasis on Whole Foods: The diet emphasizes whole, unprocessed foods such as meat, fish, poultry, eggs, non-starchy vegetables, nuts, seeds, and healthy fats like olive oil and avocado. Processed foods, sugary snacks, and refined grains are restricted or eliminated.

5. Balanced Nutrition: While carbohydrates are restricted, the diet encourages a balanced intake of nutrients, including vitamins, minerals, and fiber. This is achieved by incorporating a variety of whole foods from different food groups.

6. Customizable to Individual Needs: The Atkins Diet offers flexibility and can be customized to fit individual preferences, dietary restrictions, and lifestyle. It provides options for vegetarians, vegans, and individuals with specific dietary needs.

7. Lifestyle Changes: Beyond dietary changes, the Atkins Diet encourages adopting healthy lifestyle habits such as regular physical activity, adequate hydration, and stress management. These lifestyle factors play a crucial role in overall health and weight management.

<u>Here are some additional aspects and principles of the Atkins Diet:</u>

1. Ketosis: One of the key mechanisms of the Atkins Diet is the induction of ketosis. Ketosis occurs when the body switches from using carbohydrates as its

primary fuel source to using fat, including stored body fat and dietary fat, for energy. This metabolic state is achieved by severely limiting carbohydrate intake, typically to less than 50 grams per day during the initial phase of the diet.

2. Net Carbs: The Atkins Diet introduces the concept of "net carbs," which refers to the total carbohydrate content of a food minus the fiber content and sugar alcohols (if applicable). This approach focuses on the impact of carbohydrates on blood sugar levels, as fiber and sugar alcohols are not fully absorbed and metabolized by the body, thus having a lesser effect on blood glucose.

3. Glycemic Index (GI): While not strictly based on the glycemic index, the Atkins Diet encourages choosing carbohydrates with a lower glycemic index, which are less likely to cause rapid spikes in blood sugar levels. Foods with a lower GI include non-starchy vegetables, nuts, seeds, and certain fruits.

4. Meal Frequency: The Atkins Diet does not prescribe specific meal frequencies or timing but encourages listening to hunger cues and eating when hungry. Some individuals on the diet find success with intermittent fasting or eating smaller, more frequent meals, depending on their preferences and lifestyle.

5. Hydration: Adequate hydration is emphasized on the Atkins Diet to support overall health and weight loss. Drinking plenty of water throughout the day helps maintain hydration, supports digestion, and may help curb appetite.

6. Supplementation: The Atkins Diet recommends supplementation with vitamins, minerals, and electrolytes, especially during the initial phases when carbohydrate

intake is restricted. This helps ensure adequate nutrient intake and may prevent potential deficiencies.

7. Long-Term Maintenance: The Atkins Diet aims to provide a sustainable approach to weight loss and maintenance by gradually reintroducing carbohydrates and encouraging a balanced, whole-foods-based diet in the long term. The Maintenance Phase focuses on finding a sustainable carbohydrate intake level that supports weight maintenance while promoting overall health.

<u>History and evolution of the Atkins Diet</u>

The Atkins Diet, created by Dr. Robert Atkins, has a rich history and has evolved significantly since its inception in the 1960s.

1960s-1970s: Inception and Early Years
- Dr. Robert Atkins first introduced the Atkins Diet in the 1960s based on his observations of weight loss and improved health in patients who followed a low-carbohydrate, high-fat diet.
- In 1972, Dr. Atkins published his book "Dr. Atkins' Diet Revolution," outlining his dietary principles and approach to weight loss.
- The diet gained popularity as an alternative to traditional low-fat, calorie-restricted diets of the time.

1980s-1990s: Growth and Criticism
- Throughout the 1980s and 1990s, the Atkins Diet continued to gain popularity, with millions of people trying the program and experiencing weight loss success.

- However, the diet also faced criticism from some health experts and organizations who questioned its high-fat content and potential long-term health implications, particularly regarding cardiovascular health.

2000s: Revisions and Research
- In the early 2000s, Dr. Atkins revised and updated his original diet plan with the release of "Dr. Atkins' New Diet Revolution," which included additional phases and updated nutritional information.
- During this time, scientific research on low-carbohydrate diets, including the Atkins Diet, gained momentum, with studies suggesting their effectiveness for weight loss and metabolic health.
- The Atkins Diet underwent further modifications to address criticisms and incorporate new research findings, including emphasizing the importance of whole foods and healthy fats.

2010s-Present: Continued Evolution
- In recent years, the Atkins Diet has continued to evolve with the introduction of new products, online resources, and mobile apps to support individuals following the program.
- The diet has expanded to include various Atkins-branded products such as bars, shakes, and frozen meals, offering convenient options for followers.
- Additionally, the Atkins Diet has adapted to changing dietary trends and consumer preferences, offering flexible approaches to accommodate different lifestyles and dietary needs.
Let's delve deeper into the history and evolution of the Atkins Diet:

Scientific Research and Validation:

- Over the years, numerous scientific studies have been conducted to evaluate the efficacy and safety of the Atkins Diet and other low-carbohydrate approaches.

- Research has shown that low-carbohydrate diets, including the Atkins Diet, can lead to significant weight loss, improvements in metabolic health markers such as blood sugar levels and triglycerides, and even better adherence compared to traditional low-fat diets in some studies.

Popularity and Cultural Impact:

- The Atkins Diet has had a significant impact on popular culture and the food industry. It sparked a renewed interest in low-carbohydrate eating and influenced food trends, leading to the development of a wide range of low-carb products and menu options.

- The diet's popularity also led to the creation of numerous cookbooks, websites, and online communities dedicated to sharing Atkins-friendly recipes, meal plans, and support.

Variations and Adaptations:

- Over time, variations and adaptations of the Atkins Diet have emerged to cater to different preferences and dietary needs. These include modified versions for vegetarians, vegans, and individuals with specific health conditions such as diabetes.

- Some variations of the Atkins Diet incorporate concepts from other dietary approaches, such as Mediterranean-style eating or intermittent fasting, to provide a more comprehensive approach to health and weight management.

Criticism and Controversy:

- Despite its popularity and success stories, the Atkins Diet has also faced criticism and controversy, particularly regarding its high-fat content and potential long-term health effects.

- Critics have raised concerns about the diet's impact on cardiovascular health, cholesterol levels, and kidney function. However, research findings on these topics have been mixed, with some studies suggesting neutral or even beneficial effects on cardiovascular risk factors for some individuals.

Integration with Mainstream Nutrition:

- In recent years, elements of the Atkins Diet, such as reducing refined carbohydrates and increasing intake of whole foods and healthy fats, have been incorporated into mainstream nutrition recommendations.

- Concepts like glycemic index, net carbohydrates, and the importance of individualized dietary approaches have gained recognition and acceptance within the broader nutrition and health community.

Benefits and potential drawbacks of the Atkins Diet

The benefits and potential drawbacks of the Atkins Diet:

Benefits:

1. Weight Loss: The Atkins Diet is well-known for its effectiveness in promoting weight loss, particularly during the initial phases of carbohydrate restriction. By reducing carbohydrate intake and promoting fat burning, individuals often experience rapid weight loss, especially in the form of reduced body fat.

2. Improved Metabolic Health: Research suggests that low-carbohydrate diets like Atkins may lead to improvements in metabolic health markers such as blood sugar levels, insulin sensitivity, triglycerides, and HDL (good) cholesterol levels. This can be particularly beneficial for individuals with insulin resistance, prediabetes, or type 2 diabetes.

3. Increased Satiety: The high protein and fat content of the Atkins Diet can help increase feelings of fullness and satiety, leading to reduced appetite and overall calorie intake. This can make it easier for individuals to adhere to the diet and maintain a calorie deficit for weight loss.

4. Better Blood Sugar Control: By reducing carbohydrate intake and stabilizing blood sugar levels, the Atkins Diet may help improve blood sugar control, reducing the risk of insulin spikes and crashes commonly associated with high-carbohydrate meals.

5. Flexible and Customizable: The Atkins Diet offers various phases and options to suit individual preferences, dietary restrictions, and lifestyle. It can be adapted to accommodate vegetarians, vegans, and individuals with specific health conditions, making it a versatile and customizable dietary approach.

Potential Drawbacks:

1. Nutrient Deficiencies: Severely restricting carbohydrate-rich foods like fruits, whole grains, and certain vegetables may lead to potential deficiencies in essential nutrients such as fiber, vitamins, and minerals. It's important to carefully plan meals and consider supplementation to ensure adequate nutrient intake.

2. Initial Side Effects: Some individuals may experience temporary side effects during the initial phases of the Atkins Diet, such as fatigue, headache, dizziness, and constipation. These symptoms are often attributed to the body's adjustment to a low-carbohydrate diet and typically subside within a few days to weeks.

3. Long-Term Sustainability: While effective for short-term weight loss, some individuals may find it challenging to maintain the strict carbohydrate restriction of the Atkins Diet over the long term. Sustainability may depend on factors such as individual preferences, social situations, and lifestyle considerations.

4. Potential for Unhealthy Food Choices: While the Atkins Diet emphasizes whole, unprocessed foods, some individuals may interpret the diet as a license to consume high amounts of processed meats, saturated fats, and artificial sweeteners, which may not align with overall health recommendations.

5. Individual Variability: Like any dietary approach, the response to the Atkins Diet can vary among individuals. While some may experience significant weight loss and health improvements, others may not achieve the same results or may experience adverse effects.

Chapter 2: Getting Started with Atkins

Assessing your current diet and lifestyle

As an individual considering or currently following the Atkins Diet, it's essential to assess your current diet and lifestyle to ensure successful adoption and adherence to the program. Here's how you can assess your current habits and make adjustments to align with the principles of the Atkins Diet:

1. Evaluate Your Current Diet:

- Take a close look at your current dietary habits, including the types of foods you regularly consume and their macronutrient composition (carbohydrates, protein, and fats).

- Identify high-carbohydrate foods such as bread, pasta, rice, sugary snacks, and processed foods that may need to be reduced or eliminated on the Atkins Diet.

- Consider your intake of protein-rich foods such as meat, poultry, fish, eggs, and dairy products, as these will be emphasized on the Atkins Diet.

2. Assess Your Macronutrient Balance:

- Calculate your current intake of carbohydrates, protein, and fats to determine your baseline macronutrient balance.

- Compare your current macronutrient intake to the recommended macronutrient distribution for the Atkins Diet, which typically involves a higher proportion of fats and proteins and a lower proportion of carbohydrates, especially during the initial phases.

3. Identify Areas for Adjustment:

- Identify areas of your current diet that may need adjustment to align with the Atkins Diet principles. This may include reducing or eliminating high-carbohydrate foods, increasing intake of protein-rich foods and healthy fats, and incorporating more non-starchy vegetables.
- Consider any potential challenges or barriers to following the Atkins Diet, such as social situations, dining out, or specific food preferences, and brainstorm strategies to overcome these obstacles.

4. Evaluate Your Lifestyle Habits:
- Assess your current lifestyle habits, including physical activity level, stress management, sleep quality, and hydration status.
- Recognize the importance of regular physical activity in conjunction with the Atkins Diet for overall health, weight management, and metabolic health.
- Consider strategies to manage stress effectively, prioritize sleep hygiene, and stay adequately hydrated, as these lifestyle factors can impact your success on the Atkins Diet.

5. Set Realistic Goals and Create a Plan:
- Based on your assessment, set realistic goals for adopting the Atkins Diet, taking into account your individual preferences, health goals, and lifestyle factors.
- Create a personalized plan outlining specific dietary changes, meal planning strategies, exercise routines, and lifestyle modifications to support your success on the Atkins Diet.
- Consider tracking your progress, including changes in weight, body measurements, energy levels, and overall well-being, to monitor the effectiveness of the Atkins Diet for you personally.

6. Food Logging and Tracking:

- Consider keeping a food journal or using a mobile app to track your food intake. This can help you become more aware of your eating habits and identify areas where adjustments are needed to align with the Atkins Diet.
- Pay attention to portion sizes and serving sizes of different foods, as portion control plays a crucial role in managing calorie intake and macronutrient balance.

7. Mindful Eating:

- Practice mindful eating by paying attention to hunger and fullness cues, as well as the sensory experience of eating. This can help you make more conscious food choices and avoid overeating.
- Slow down during meals, chew food thoroughly, and savor each bite to enhance satisfaction and reduce the tendency to overeat.

8. Social Support and Accountability:

- Seek support from friends, family members, or online communities following the Atkins Diet. Having a support system can provide encouragement, motivation, and accountability throughout your journey.
- Consider joining local or online support groups, forums, or social media communities where you can connect with others who are also following the Atkins Diet for mutual support and sharing experiences.

9. Education and Resources:

- Take advantage of educational resources, including books, websites, and online tools provided by Atkins Nutritionals or other reputable sources. These resources can offer guidance on meal planning, recipes, grocery shopping, and navigating social situations while following the Atkins Diet.

- Stay informed about the latest research and developments related to low-carbohydrate diets and their potential impact on health and weight management.

10. Regular Monitoring and Adjustments:

- Monitor your progress regularly by tracking key indicators such as weight, body measurements, blood sugar levels (if applicable), energy levels, and overall well-being.

- Be prepared to make adjustments to your diet and lifestyle as needed based on your progress and feedback from your body. This may involve fine-tuning your macronutrient balance, adjusting portion sizes, or incorporating new strategies to overcome challenges.

<u>Setting realistic goals as an Atkins Diet patient</u>

Setting realistic goals as an Atkins Diet patient is crucial for success and long-term adherence to the diet. Here are some key steps to setting achievable goals:

1. Understand the Diet: Before setting goals, ensure you have a clear understanding of the Atkins Diet, its phases, allowed foods, and recommended portions. This will help you set realistic expectations.

2. Consult a Healthcare Professional: Speak with a healthcare professional or a registered dietitian who can provide personalized guidance based on your health status, goals, and any medical conditions you may have.

3. Set Specific Goals: Instead of setting vague goals like "lose weight," be specific. For example, aim to lose a certain number of pounds within a realistic timeframe.

4. Be Realistic: Set goals that are achievable based on your lifestyle, commitments, and the recommendations of your healthcare provider. Unrealistic goals can lead to frustration and discouragement.

5. Consider Non-Scale Victories: While weight loss is often a primary goal, consider other markers of progress such as improved energy levels, better sleep, or fitting into smaller clothing sizes.

6. Break Down Goals: If your ultimate goal is significant, break it down into smaller, more manageable goals. For example, if you aim to lose 50 pounds, set milestones to celebrate every 5 or 10-pound loss.

7. Track Progress: Keep track of your food intake, exercise, and progress towards your goals. This can be done through a journal, app, or with the help of a healthcare professional.

8. Adjust as Needed: Be flexible and willing to adjust your goals as you progress. If you reach a plateau or encounter challenges, reassess and modify your goals accordingly.

9. Celebrate Achievements: Celebrate your successes along the way, whether it's reaching a milestone, sticking to the diet during social events, or making healthier food choices.

10. Focus on Long-Term Health: Remember that the Atkins Diet is not just about short-term weight loss but also about improving overall health and wellness. Focus on making sustainable lifestyle changes for long-term success.

Let's delve deeper into setting realistic goals as an Atkins diet patient:

1. Understanding Macronutrients: The Atkins Diet focuses on controlling carbohydrate intake while prioritizing protein and healthy fats. Set goals related to your macronutrient ratios, aiming to stay within the recommended carbohydrate limits for each phase of the diet.

2. Meal Planning and Preparation: Set goals related to meal planning and preparation to ensure you have nutritious, Atkins-friendly meals readily available. This could involve setting aside time each week to plan your meals, grocery shop for appropriate ingredients, and prep meals in advance to avoid relying on convenience foods.

3. Hydration: Adequate hydration is important for overall health and can support weight loss on the Atkins Diet. Set goals to drink a certain amount of water each day, aiming for at least eight glasses or more depending on your individual needs and activity level.

4. Physical Activity: While the Atkins Diet primarily focuses on dietary changes, incorporating regular physical activity can enhance weight loss and overall health. Set realistic goals related to physical activity, such as aiming for a certain number of minutes of exercise each week or incorporating daily movement breaks into your routine.

5. Stress Management: Stress can impact weight loss and overall well-being. Set goals related to stress management techniques such as mindfulness, meditation, deep breathing exercises, or engaging in activities that bring you joy and relaxation.

6. Sleep Quality: Adequate sleep is essential for weight loss and overall health. Set goals related to improving sleep quality and quantity, aiming for 7-9 hours of uninterrupted sleep each night and establishing a consistent bedtime routine.

7. Monitoring Progress: Regularly monitor your progress towards your goals to stay motivated and identify areas for improvement. This could involve tracking your food intake, physical activity, weight, measurements, and other relevant health metrics.

8. Seek Support: Don't hesitate to seek support from healthcare professionals, online communities, friends, or family members who can provide encouragement, accountability, and guidance throughout your Atkins Diet journey.

9. Adherence to Phases: The Atkins Diet consists of different phases, each with specific guidelines and carbohydrate levels. Set goals to adhere to the recommendations of each phase, gradually transitioning through the phases as directed to maximize results.

10. Mindful Eating: Practice mindful eating techniques to enhance awareness of hunger and fullness cues, prevent overeating, and foster a healthier relationship

with food. Set goals related to mindful eating practices such as eating slowly, savoring each bite, and avoiding distractions during meals.

<u>Understanding the four phases of the Atkins Diet</u>

The Atkins Diet is a low-carbohydrate diet that consists of four phases designed to promote weight loss, improve metabolic health, and support long-term wellness. Each phase has specific guidelines regarding carbohydrate intake, food choices, and duration. Let's explore each phase in detail:

1. Phase 1: Induction Phase (Atkins 20) / Phase 1: Kickstart (Atkins 40):

   - Objective: The primary goal of the induction phase is to kickstart weight loss by transitioning the body into a state of ketosis, where it burns fat for fuel instead of carbohydrates.

   - Duration: Typically lasts for two weeks, but can vary depending on individual goals and metabolic responses.

   - Carbohydrate Intake: Very limited carbohydrate intake, usually around 20-25 grams of net carbs per day for Atkins 20, and 40 grams of net carbs per day for Atkins 40.

   - Allowed Foods: Focus on high-protein foods, healthy fats, and non-starchy vegetables. Common foods include meat, poultry, fish, eggs, cheese, nuts, seeds, oils, and low-carb vegetables such as leafy greens, broccoli, and cauliflower.

- Foods to Avoid: High-carb foods such as grains, sugars, starchy vegetables, fruits, and processed foods are restricted during this phase.

- Hydration: Adequate hydration is encouraged, including water, herbal tea, and sugar-free beverages.

- Supplements: Some individuals may benefit from taking electrolyte supplements to prevent electrolyte imbalances during the initial phase of carbohydrate restriction.

- Potential Side Effects: Some individuals may experience side effects during the induction phase, often referred to as the "keto flu," including fatigue, headache, dizziness, and irritability. These symptoms typically subside as the body adapts to using fat for fuel.

2. Phase 2: Ongoing Weight Loss (OWL):

- Objective: The ongoing weight loss phase focuses on gradual weight loss while expanding food choices and increasing carbohydrate intake slightly.

- Duration: This phase continues until you are within 10 pounds of your goal weight.

- Carbohydrate Intake: Gradual increase in carbohydrate intake, usually adding 5 grams of net carbs per week, with the aim of finding your personal carb tolerance level for continued weight loss.

- Allowed Foods: In addition to foods allowed in Phase 1, you can gradually introduce small amounts of fruits, certain whole grains, and legumes back into your diet while monitoring their impact on weight loss and ketosis.

- Portion Control: Emphasis on portion control and mindful eating to support continued weight loss and prevent overeating.

- Monitoring Progress: Regularly monitor your weight, measurements, and how your body responds to increased carbohydrate intake to determine your individual tolerance level.

3. Phase 3: Pre-Maintenance:

- Objective: The pre-maintenance phase prepares you for long-term weight maintenance by further increasing carbohydrate intake while continuing to monitor portion sizes and food choices.

- Duration: Typically lasts until you reach your goal weight and maintain it for at least a month.

- Carbohydrate Intake: Gradual increase in carbohydrate intake, usually adding 10 grams of net carbs per week, focusing on nutrient-dense, whole-food sources of carbohydrates.

- Reintroducing Carbohydrates: Experiment with reintroducing additional carbohydrate sources such as whole grains, fruits, and starchy vegetables while monitoring their impact on weight maintenance and overall well-being.

- Transition to Maintenance: Use this phase to transition from a weight loss-focused mindset to a maintenance-focused approach, emphasizing sustainable dietary habits and lifestyle changes.

4. Phase 4: Maintenance:

- Objective: The maintenance phase focuses on sustaining your weight loss and overall health by adopting a balanced, long-term approach to eating and lifestyle.

- Duration: This phase is ongoing and becomes a permanent way of eating to support weight maintenance and optimal health.

- Carbohydrate Intake: Gradually increase carbohydrate intake to a level that allows you to maintain your weight and energy levels while still prioritizing nutrient-dense, whole-food sources of carbohydrates.

- Balanced Diet: Emphasis on consuming a balanced diet that includes a variety of foods from all food groups, including carbohydrates, proteins, healthy fats, fruits, vegetables, and whole grains.

- Portion Control and Moderation: Continue practicing portion control, mindful eating, and moderation to prevent weight regain and promote overall health and well-being.

- Regular Monitoring: Regularly monitor your weight, measurements, and overall health markers to ensure you are maintaining your desired weight and making adjustments as needed.

Chapter 3: Phase 1: Induction

Overview of Phase 1

Phase 1 of the Atkins Diet, also known as the Induction Phase, is the initial stage designed to kickstart weight loss by transitioning the body into a state of ketosis. Ketosis is a metabolic state where the body burns fat for fuel instead of carbohydrates, resulting in increased fat burning and rapid weight loss for many individuals. Here's a detailed overview of Phase 1:

1. Objective:

   - The primary goal of Phase 1 is to induce ketosis and initiate rapid weight loss by severely restricting carbohydrate intake.

2. Duration:

   - Phase 1 typically lasts for two weeks, but the duration may vary depending on individual goals, metabolic responses, and adherence to the diet plan.

3. Carbohydrate Intake:

   - Carbohydrate intake is severely restricted during Phase 1, usually limited to around 20-25 grams of net carbs per day for Atkins 20, and 40 grams of net carbs per day for Atkins 40.
   - Net carbs are calculated by subtracting fiber and sugar alcohols from the total carbohydrate content of foods, as they have a minimal impact on blood sugar levels.

4. Allowed Foods:

- Phase 1 emphasizes high-protein foods, healthy fats, and non-starchy vegetables, while restricting high-carbohydrate foods.

  - Allowed foods include:

  - Protein sources: Meat, poultry, fish, seafood, eggs.

  - High-fat dairy: Cheese, butter, cream.

  - Healthy fats: Olive oil, coconut oil, avocado oil.

  - Non-starchy vegetables: Leafy greens (spinach, kale, lettuce), broccoli, cauliflower, zucchini, cucumbers, bell peppers, asparagus, mushrooms, etc.

  - Herbs, spices, and condiments: Salt, pepper, garlic, herbs, vinegar, mustard, mayonnaise (sugar-free), soy sauce (low-sodium).

5. Foods to Avoid:

  - High-carbohydrate foods are restricted during Phase 1 to induce ketosis and promote rapid weight loss. Foods to avoid include:

  - Grains: Bread, pasta, rice, cereal, oats.

  - Sugars: Table sugar, honey, maple syrup, agave nectar, desserts, candy, sugary beverages.

  - Starchy vegetables: Potatoes, sweet potatoes, corn, peas, winter squash.

  - Fruits: Bananas, apples, oranges, grapes, mangoes, pineapple, dried fruits.

  - Processed foods: Packaged snacks, chips, cookies, crackers, sugary sauces and dressings.

6. Hydration:

  - Adequate hydration is essential during Phase 1 to support metabolic processes and prevent dehydration, especially as the body adjusts to using fat for fuel.

  - Drink plenty of water throughout the day, and consider incorporating herbal tea, sugar-free beverages, and electrolyte-rich fluids if needed.

7. Supplements:

- Some individuals may benefit from taking electrolyte supplements during Phase 1 to prevent electrolyte imbalances and alleviate symptoms of the "keto flu," such as fatigue, headache, dizziness, and muscle cramps.

8. Portion Control:

- While there are no strict portion control guidelines in Phase 1, it's essential to listen to your body's hunger and fullness cues and avoid overeating, especially high-calorie foods.

9. Monitoring Progress:

- Monitor your weight, measurements, and how your body responds to the diet during Phase 1 to assess progress and adjust as needed.

- Keep track of your food intake, carbohydrate consumption, and any symptoms or changes in energy levels or well-being.

10. Transitioning to Phase 2:

- After completing Phase 1, individuals can transition to Phase 2 (Ongoing Weight Loss) by gradually increasing carbohydrate intake while continuing to focus on weight loss goals and healthy eating habits.

Let's delve deeper into Phase 1 of the Atkins Diet:

1. Understanding Ketosis:

- Ketosis is a metabolic state where the body shifts from using carbohydrates as its primary fuel source to using fat for energy. This occurs when carbohydrate intake is severely restricted, leading the body to produce ketones from fat stores as an alternative fuel source.

2. Benefits of Ketosis:

   - Inducing ketosis during Phase 1 of the Atkins Diet offers several potential benefits, including:

   - Rapid weight loss: By burning fat for fuel, the body can efficiently utilize stored fat reserves, leading to significant weight loss, particularly in the form of body fat.

   - Appetite suppression: Ketosis has been associated with reduced appetite and cravings, which can make it easier to adhere to a calorie-restricted diet and achieve weight loss goals.

   - Improved metabolic markers: Ketosis may lead to improvements in metabolic health markers such as blood sugar levels, insulin sensitivity, triglycerides, and HDL cholesterol levels.

   - Increased energy and mental clarity: Some individuals report experiencing increased energy levels and mental clarity while in ketosis, which can enhance overall well-being and productivity.

3. Managing Ketosis:

   - Achieving and maintaining ketosis requires strict adherence to the carbohydrate restriction guidelines of Phase 1. To ensure success:

   - Monitor carbohydrate intake: Keep track of net carbohydrate intake from all foods and beverages consumed throughout the day, aiming to stay within the recommended limits.

   - Choose low-carb foods: Focus on consuming foods that are naturally low in carbohydrates, such as protein-rich meats, fish, eggs, and non-starchy vegetables.

- Read food labels: Pay attention to the carbohydrate content of packaged foods and ingredients to avoid hidden sources of carbohydrates.

- Test ketone levels: Some individuals may choose to monitor their ketone levels using urine strips, blood ketone meters, or breath ketone analyzers to confirm ketosis.

4. Addressing Potential Challenges:

- While ketosis can be an effective strategy for weight loss, some individuals may experience challenges or side effects during Phase 1, including:

- Keto flu: Common symptoms experienced during the initial transition to ketosis include fatigue, headache, dizziness, irritability, and muscle cramps. These symptoms are often temporary and can be alleviated by staying hydrated, replenishing electrolytes, and ensuring adequate rest.

- Social situations: Adhering to a low-carb diet may require navigating social situations and dining out while avoiding high-carbohydrate foods. Planning ahead, communicating your dietary needs to others, and making smart food choices can help you stay on track.

- Individual responses: It's essential to recognize that individual responses to ketosis may vary. While some individuals may thrive on a low-carb, ketogenic diet, others may find it challenging to sustain long-term or may experience adverse effects. Listening to your body, consulting with a healthcare professional, and making adjustments as needed are key.

5. Transitioning Out of Phase 1:

- After completing Phase 1 of the Atkins Diet, individuals can transition to Phase 2 (Ongoing Weight Loss) by gradually increasing carbohydrate intake while continuing to focus on weight loss goals and healthy eating habits. This transition allows for greater dietary flexibility while still promoting continued weight loss and metabolic health improvements.

<u>Acceptable foods and portion sizes for Atkins diet patient</u>

For an Atkins diet patient, acceptable foods typically include:

- Protein sources: Meat (beef, pork, lamb, poultry, etc.), fish, seafood, eggs, tofu, tempeh.

- Low-carb vegetables: Leafy greens (spinach, kale, lettuce), cruciferous vegetables (broccoli, cauliflower, cabbage), peppers, zucchini, mushrooms.

- Healthy fats: Avocado, olive oil, coconut oil, nuts (in moderation), seeds (chia, flaxseed, pumpkin seeds).

- Dairy: Full-fat cheese, butter, cream, plain Greek yogurt (in moderation).

- Beverages: Water, herbal tea, coffee (in moderation).

Let's delve deeper into acceptable foods and portion sizes for someone following the Atkins diet:

1. Protein Sources:
   - Aim for high-quality protein sources such as:
     - Beef
     - Pork
     - Lamb
     - Poultry (chicken, turkey)
     - Fish (salmon, trout, tuna, mackerel)
     - Seafood (shrimp, crab, lobster)
     - Eggs
     - Tofu

- Tempeh

- Portion sizes: Typically 3-6 ounces (85-170 grams) of cooked protein per meal. Adjust based on individual needs and goals.

2. Low-Carb Vegetables:

- Focus on non-starchy vegetables that are low in carbohydrates and high in fiber. Some examples include:

- Leafy greens (spinach, kale, lettuce)

- Cruciferous vegetables (broccoli, cauliflower, cabbage)

- Bell peppers

- Zucchini

- Mushrooms

- Asparagus

- Green beans

- Portion sizes: Aim for 1-2 cups (approximately 100-200 grams) of cooked vegetables per meal. Adjust based on individual preferences and tolerance.

3. Healthy Fats:

- Include sources of healthy fats to promote satiety and support overall health. Examples include:

- Avocado

- Olive oil

- Coconut oil

- Butter (preferably grass-fed)

- Full-fat cheese

- Nuts (almonds, walnuts, pecans) and seeds (chia seeds, flaxseeds, pumpkin seeds)

- Portion sizes: Practice moderation with fats, as they are calorie-dense. Aim for appropriate serving sizes based on individual calorie and macronutrient needs.

4. Dairy:
   - Choose full-fat or low-carb dairy options:
     - Full-fat cheese
     - Butter
     - Cream
     - Plain Greek yogurt (preferably full-fat and unsweetened)

- Portion sizes: Moderate intake based on individual tolerance to lactose and calorie goals. Opt for plain varieties without added sugars.

5. Beverages:
   - Stay hydrated with low-carb beverage options such as:
     - Water
     - Herbal tea (unsweetened)
     - Coffee (black or with minimal added cream or sweeteners, if desired)

- Avoid sugary beverages, including soda, fruit juice, and sweetened coffee drinks.

Portion sizes on the Atkins diet can vary depending on the phase of the diet and individual needs, but generally, protein portions should be around 3-6 ounces per meal, and vegetable servings should be around 1-2 cups per meal.

<u>Tips for overcoming carb cravings for an Atkins diet patient</u>

Here are some tips to help overcome carb cravings for someone following the Atkins diet:

1. Stay Hydrated: Drink plenty of water throughout the day. Sometimes, thirst can be mistaken for hunger or cravings.

2. Include Protein in Every Meal: Protein helps promote satiety and can help reduce cravings for carbohydrates. Incorporate lean protein sources like chicken, fish, tofu, or eggs into your meals.

3. Choose Healthy Fats: Including healthy fats in your meals can help keep you feeling full and satisfied. Opt for sources like avocado, olive oil, nuts, and seeds.

4. Eat Regularly: Aim to eat regular meals and snacks throughout the day to keep your blood sugar levels stable and reduce the likelihood of cravings.

5. Focus on Low-Carb Vegetables: Fill up on non-starchy vegetables, which are low in carbs and high in fiber. They can help keep you feeling full and satisfied without spiking your blood sugar levels.

6. Plan Ahead: Plan your meals and snacks in advance to ensure you have low-carb options readily available. This can help prevent impulsive carb cravings.

7. Practice Mindful Eating: Pay attention to your hunger and fullness cues. Eat slowly and savor each bite, which can help prevent overeating and reduce cravings.

8. Find Low-Carb Alternatives: Look for low-carb alternatives to your favorite carb-rich foods. For example, cauliflower rice or zucchini noodles can be substituted for rice or pasta.

9. Stay Busy: Keep yourself occupied with activities or hobbies to distract yourself from cravings. Physical activity can also help reduce cravings and improve mood.

10. Seek Support: Reach out to friends, family, or a support group for encouragement and accountability. Having someone to share your journey with can help keep you motivated and on track.

11. Include Fiber-Rich Foods: Foods high in fiber, such as leafy greens, nuts, seeds, and low-carb vegetables, can help you feel fuller for longer and reduce cravings for carbs.

12. Limit Artificial Sweeteners: While some artificial sweeteners are low in carbs and can be included in moderation, they may trigger cravings for sweet foods in some individuals. Consider limiting or avoiding them if you find they increase your cravings.

13. Practice Stress Management: Stress can trigger cravings for high-carb foods. Incorporate stress-relief techniques such as deep breathing, meditation, yoga, or going for a walk to help manage stress and reduce cravings.

14. Get Enough Sleep: Lack of sleep can disrupt hunger hormones and increase cravings for carbs. Aim for seven to nine hours of quality sleep each night to support overall health and reduce cravings.

15. Address Emotional Eating: Identify any emotional triggers that may lead to carb cravings, such as boredom, sadness, or stress. Find alternative ways to cope with emotions, such as journaling, talking to a friend, or engaging in a hobby.

16. Experiment with Intermittent Fasting: Some individuals find that intermittent fasting, where meals are consumed within a specific time window each day, can help reduce cravings and improve insulin sensitivity. Consult with a healthcare professional before trying intermittent fasting.

17. Stay Consistent: Consistency is key when following the Atkins diet. Stick to your meal plan and avoid deviating from your chosen food options to help minimize cravings and maintain ketosis (if applicable).

18. Stay Educated: Learn about the science behind the Atkins diet and how it affects your body. Understanding the metabolic changes that occur when following a low-carb diet can help reinforce your commitment and reduce cravings.

19. Reward Yourself: Set non-food-related rewards for yourself when you successfully overcome carb cravings or reach milestones on your Atkins diet journey. This can help reinforce positive behavior and motivate you to stay on track.

20. Seek Professional Support: If you're struggling to overcome carb cravings or adhere to the Atkins diet, consider seeking support from a registered dietitian, nutritionist, or healthcare professional who can provide personalized guidance and support.

<u>Sample meal plans and recipes</u>

Here are sample meal plans and recipes for someone following the Atkins diet:

Sample Meal Plan 1: Induction Phase

Breakfast:
- Scrambled eggs with spinach and mushrooms cooked in olive oil
- Side of avocado slices
- Herbal tea or black coffee

Lunch:
- Grilled chicken breast with mixed greens (lettuce, cucumber, bell peppers)
- Olive oil and vinegar dressing
- Snack: Celery sticks with cream cheese

Dinner:
- Baked salmon with garlic butter sauce
- Steamed broccoli
- Side salad with mixed greens and ranch dressing
- Snack: Handful of almonds

Sample Meal Plan 2: Balancing Phase

Breakfast:

- Greek yogurt with mixed berries and chopped nuts

- Side of scrambled eggs

- Herbal tea or black coffee

Lunch:

- Grilled shrimp Caesar salad with romaine lettuce, Parmesan cheese, and Caesar dressing

- Snack: Sliced cucumber with guacamole

Dinner:

- Zucchini noodles with pesto sauce and grilled chicken

- Side of sautéed spinach

- Snack: Cheese and turkey roll-ups

Sample Meal Plan 3: Pre-Maintenance Phase

Breakfast:

- Spinach and feta omelet

- Side of avocado slices

- Herbal tea or black coffee

Lunch:

- Turkey and avocado lettuce wraps with mayonnaise

- Side of mixed greens with olive oil and vinegar dressing

- Snack: Celery sticks with almond butter

Dinner:

- Grilled steak with garlic butter

- Cauliflower mashed "potatoes"

- Side of roasted Brussels sprouts

- Snack: Greek yogurt with a drizzle of honey

Sample Atkins-Friendly Recipes:

1. Cauliflower Fried Rice:

   - Ingredients: Cauliflower rice, diced vegetables (bell peppers, onions, carrots), scrambled eggs, soy sauce (or tamari for gluten-free), sesame oil, garlic, ginger.

   - Instructions: Sauté diced vegetables in sesame oil with minced garlic and ginger. Add cauliflower rice and cook until tender. Push the mixture to one side of the pan and scramble eggs on the other side. Mix everything together and add soy sauce to taste.

2. Grilled Lemon Herb Chicken:

   - Ingredients: Chicken breasts, lemon juice, olive oil, garlic, herbs (such as thyme, rosemary, parsley), salt, pepper.

   - Instructions: Marinate chicken breasts in a mixture of lemon juice, olive oil, minced garlic, chopped herbs, salt, and pepper for at least 30 minutes. Grill until cooked through and juicy.

3. Zucchini Noodles with Pesto Sauce:

   - Ingredients: Zucchini noodles (zoodles), homemade or store-bought pesto sauce, cherry tomatoes, grated Parmesan cheese.

- Instructions: Sauté zucchini noodles in a skillet until tender. Toss with pesto sauce and halved cherry tomatoes. Top with grated Parmesan cheese before serving.

4. Crispy Baked Parmesan Zucchini Fries:
   - Ingredients: Zucchini, grated Parmesan cheese, almond flour (or coconut flour), eggs, salt, pepper, garlic powder.
   - Instructions: Cut zucchini into fries. Dip in beaten eggs, then coat with a mixture of grated Parmesan cheese, almond flour, salt, pepper, and garlic powder. Place on a baking sheet lined with parchment paper and bake until crispy.

Sample Meal Plan 4: Maintenance Phase

Breakfast:
- Omelet with mushrooms, bell peppers, and feta cheese
- Side of sliced tomatoes
- Herbal tea or black coffee

Lunch:
- Grilled salmon with a lemon dill sauce
- Caesar salad with romaine lettuce, bacon, and Parmesan cheese
- Snack: Cucumber slices with tzatziki

Dinner:
- Beef stir-fry with broccoli, bell peppers, and snap peas in a low-carb stir-fry sauce
- Side of cauliflower rice

- Snack: Mixed berries with whipped cream

Sample Meal Plan 5: Low-Carb Snack Ideas

1. Cheese and Pepperoni Platter:
   - Ingredients: Assorted cheeses (cheddar, mozzarella, etc.), pepperoni slices, cherry tomatoes, olives.
   - Instructions: Arrange cheese and pepperoni on a platter with cherry tomatoes and olives for a satisfying and low-carb snack.

2. Spicy Guacamole with Veggie Sticks:
   - Ingredients: Avocado, tomatoes, onions, cilantro, lime juice, jalapeño (optional), assorted vegetable sticks (cucumber, bell peppers, celery).
   - Instructions: Mash avocados and mix with diced tomatoes, onions, cilantro, lime juice, and jalapeño for a spicy guacamole. Serve with vegetable sticks for dipping.

3. Hard-Boiled Eggs with Salt and Pepper:
   - Ingredients: Hard-boiled eggs, salt, pepper.
   - Instructions: Simply peel hard-boiled eggs and season with a sprinkle of salt and pepper for a quick and protein-rich snack.

4. Caprese Skewers:
   - Ingredients: Cherry tomatoes, fresh mozzarella balls, basil leaves, balsamic glaze.
   - Instructions: Thread cherry tomatoes, fresh mozzarella balls, and basil leaves onto skewers. Drizzle with balsamic glaze for a tasty and low-carb appetizer.

Low-Carb Recipes:

1. Cauliflower Pizza Crust:

  - Ingredients: Cauliflower rice, egg, mozzarella cheese, Italian seasoning, salt.

  - Instructions: Mix cauliflower rice with egg, mozzarella cheese, Italian seasoning, and salt. Press into a crust shape and bake until golden. Add desired pizza toppings and bake until cheese is melted.

2. Lettuce Wrap Tacos:

  - Ingredients: Ground beef or turkey, taco seasoning, lettuce leaves, diced tomatoes, shredded cheese, sour cream.

  - Instructions: Brown ground beef or turkey with taco seasoning. Spoon into lettuce leaves and top with diced tomatoes, shredded cheese, and a dollop of sour cream.

3. Avocado and Bacon Stuffed Eggs:

  - Ingredients: Hard-boiled eggs, avocado, cooked bacon, mayonnaise, mustard, salt, pepper.

  - Instructions: Cut hard-boiled eggs in half and remove yolks. Mash yolks with avocado, cooked bacon, mayonnaise, mustard, salt, and pepper. Spoon mixture back into egg whites.

4. Chicken and Broccoli Alfredo:

  - Ingredients: Chicken breast, broccoli, Alfredo sauce (made with cream, Parmesan cheese, garlic), salt, pepper, olive oil.

- Instructions: Cook chicken breast and broccoli. Mix with homemade Alfredo sauce made from cream, Parmesan cheese, and garlic. Serve over cauliflower rice.

These sample meal plans and recipes provide a variety of options for someone following the Atkins diet, whether they're in the induction, balancing, or pre-maintenance phase.

Chapter 4: Phase 2: Ongoing Weight Loss (OWL)

Transitioning from Phase 1 to Phase 2

Transitioning from Phase 1 to Phase 2 of the Atkins diet involves gradually reintroducing carbohydrates into your meal plan while monitoring your body's response. In Phase 1, also known as the "Induction Phase," you've been consuming minimal carbs to kickstart ketosis and initiate weight loss. As you move into Phase 2, it's essential to follow the guidelines to ensure a smooth transition:

1. Gradual Introduction of Carbohydrates: Start by adding small amounts of carbohydrates to your meals, such as berries, nuts, seeds, and certain vegetables. Monitor your body's response, paying attention to any changes in weight, energy levels, or cravings.

2. Monitor Your Carb Tolerance: Each person's carb tolerance varies, so pay attention to how your body reacts to different types and amounts of carbohydrates. Some individuals may be able to tolerate more carbs than others without disrupting ketosis or weight loss progress.

3. Continue Protein and Fat Intake: While increasing your carbohydrate intake, maintain adequate protein and fat intake to support satiety and muscle preservation. Lean proteins and healthy fats should still comprise a significant portion of your meals.

4. Stay Hydrated: Drinking plenty of water is essential throughout all phases of the Atkins diet. It helps with digestion, supports metabolism, and can help alleviate cravings.

5. Regular Monitoring: Keep track of your progress by monitoring your weight, energy levels, and overall well-being. Adjust your carbohydrate intake as needed based on your individual response.

6. Incorporate Healthy Carbohydrates: Focus on incorporating nutrient-dense, high-fiber carbohydrates into your meals, such as whole grains, legumes, and additional fruits and vegetables. These sources provide essential vitamins, minerals, and fiber while minimizing blood sugar spikes.

7. Maintain a Balanced Lifestyle: Remember that the Atkins diet is not just about carb restriction but also emphasizes overall lifestyle changes, including regular physical activity and stress management.

8. Consult with a Healthcare Professional: Before making any significant dietary changes, especially if you have underlying health conditions or concerns, it's important to consult with a healthcare professional or registered dietitian who can provide personalized guidance and support.

9. Understanding Phase 2 Goals: The primary goal of Phase 2 is to continue losing weight or maintain your current weight while gradually expanding your food choices. This phase is often referred to as the "Balancing Phase" because it focuses on finding the right balance of carbohydrates for your body while still promoting fat burning.

10. Incremental Carb Increase: During Phase 2, you will gradually increase your daily carbohydrate intake by approximately 5 grams per week. This slow increase

allows you to identify your personal carbohydrate threshold without risking weight regain or disrupting ketosis abruptly.

11. Choosing the Right Carbohydrates: Not all carbohydrates are created equal. In Phase 2, focus on incorporating complex carbohydrates that are high in fiber and low in sugar to support stable blood sugar levels and sustained energy throughout the day. Examples include whole grains like quinoa, brown rice, oats, and starchy vegetables like sweet potatoes and butternut squash.

12. Monitoring Ketosis: As you increase your carbohydrate intake, you may naturally shift out of ketosis. This is normal and expected during Phase 2 of the Atkins diet. However, if your primary goal is to remain in ketosis for therapeutic reasons or continued weight loss, you may need to adjust your carbohydrate intake accordingly.

13. Listening to Your Body: Pay attention to how your body responds to the reintroduction of carbohydrates. Some individuals may find that they feel more energetic with a slightly higher carb intake, while others may prefer to stay in a lower carb range for optimal results. Adjust your carbohydrate intake based on your energy levels, cravings, and overall well-being.

14. Flexibility and Adaptability: The Atkins diet emphasizes flexibility and adaptability to accommodate individual preferences and lifestyle factors. Experiment with different food choices and meal patterns to find what works best for you in Phase 2.

15. Long-Term Maintenance: Phase 2 sets the foundation for long-term weight management and overall health. Once you've identified your carbohydrate tolerance and reached your desired weight, you can transition to Phase 3, also known as the "Pre-Maintenance Phase," where you further fine-tune your carbohydrate intake and continue practicing healthy eating habits.

<u>Expanding food choices while maintaining ketosis</u>

Expanding food choices while maintaining ketosis as an Atkins diet patient involves strategically incorporating a wider variety of low-carb, high-fat foods into your meals while monitoring your carbohydrate intake to stay within ketosis. Here are some key strategies to help you achieve this:

1. Focus on Low-Carb Vegetables**: While some vegetables are restricted in the initial phases of the Atkins diet, you can gradually expand your options as you progress. Focus on non-starchy vegetables such as leafy greens, broccoli, cauliflower, zucchini, and bell peppers, which are low in carbohydrates and high in fiber, vitamins, and minerals.

2. Incorporate Healthy Fats: Healthy fats are a cornerstone of the Atkins diet and play a crucial role in maintaining ketosis. Incorporate a variety of sources such as avocados, nuts, seeds, olive oil, coconut oil, and fatty fish like salmon and mackerel into your meals to increase flavor and satiety.

3. Choose Quality Proteins: Opt for high-quality proteins such as lean meats, poultry, eggs, and seafood to support muscle maintenance and satiety while keeping carbohydrate intake in check. Avoid processed meats and opt for grass-fed, pasture-raised, or wild-caught options whenever possible.

4. Experiment with Low-Carb Substitutes: Explore low-carb substitutes for your favorite high-carb foods to expand your meal options while staying in ketosis. For example, cauliflower rice or zucchini noodles can replace traditional rice or pasta, and almond flour or coconut flour can be used in place of wheat flour for baking.

5. Monitor Portion Sizes: While certain foods may be low in carbohydrates, consuming them in large quantities can still impact ketosis. Pay attention to portion sizes and track your carbohydrate intake to ensure you're staying within your individualized carb tolerance.

6. Read Labels and Ingredients: Be mindful of hidden carbohydrates in packaged foods and condiments. Always read labels and ingredients lists to identify any hidden sugars or starches that could potentially impact ketosis.

7. Stay Hydrated: Adequate hydration is essential for maintaining ketosis and supporting overall health. Drink plenty of water throughout the day, and consider incorporating electrolyte-rich beverages like broth or electrolyte supplements to replenish electrolytes lost through ketosis.

8. Regular Physical Activity: Engage in regular physical activity to support ketosis, improve metabolic flexibility, and enhance overall well-being. Incorporate a mix of cardiovascular exercise, strength training, and flexibility exercises into your routine to maximize benefits.

9. Diversify Your Protein Sources: While animal proteins are commonly emphasized on the Atkins diet, don't forget to include plant-based protein sources

as well. Incorporate foods like tofu, tempeh, seitan, and plant-based protein powders to add variety to your meals while keeping carbohydrates low.

10. Explore Dairy Options: Dairy products can be included in moderation on the Atkins diet, but it's important to choose full-fat, low-carb options. Experiment with different types of cheese, Greek yogurt, and heavy cream to add flavor and richness to your meals while staying within your carb limit.

11. Include Herbs and Spices: Enhance the flavor of your meals without adding extra carbohydrates by incorporating herbs, spices, and seasoning blends. Experiment with different flavor combinations to keep your meals interesting and satisfying.

12. Mindful Snacking: While snacking is not encouraged on the Atkins diet, there are still low-carb options available for when hunger strikes between meals. Opt for snacks like nuts, seeds, olives, cheese, hard-boiled eggs, or vegetable sticks with guacamole or hummus to keep you satisfied while maintaining ketosis.

13. Plan Ahead: Planning your meals and snacks in advance can help you stay on track with your carbohydrate intake while still enjoying a variety of foods. Consider meal prepping on weekends or creating a weekly meal plan to ensure you have low-carb options readily available throughout the week.

14. Get Creative with Recipes: There are countless keto-friendly recipes available online that cater to a wide range of tastes and preferences. Explore different cuisines and cooking techniques to keep your meals exciting and satisfying while adhering to the principles of the Atkins diet.

15. Mindful Eating: Practice mindful eating by paying attention to hunger and fullness cues, savoring each bite, and eating slowly to prevent overeating. This can help you maintain ketosis while still enjoying your meals and feeling satisfied.

16. Seek Support: Joining online communities or support groups dedicated to the Atkins diet or ketogenic lifestyle can provide valuable resources, recipe ideas, and encouragement from others who are also navigating the challenges of maintaining ketosis while expanding food choices.

<u>Monitoring progress and adjusting carbohydrate intake</u>

As an Atkins diet patient, monitoring your progress and adjusting your carbohydrate intake is crucial for achieving and maintaining ketosis while optimizing your weight loss or health goals. Here's how you can effectively monitor your progress and make necessary adjustments:

1. Regular Weigh-Ins: Weigh yourself regularly, ideally once a week, at the same time of day and under consistent conditions. This will help you track changes in your weight and assess the effectiveness of your current carbohydrate intake.

2. Keep a Food Journal: Record everything you eat and drink, including portion sizes and carbohydrate counts, in a food journal or using a mobile app. This will help you become more aware of your carbohydrate intake and identify any patterns or trends that may affect ketosis.

3. Monitor Ketone Levels: Use ketone testing strips or a blood ketone meter to monitor your ketone levels regularly. This will provide objective feedback on

whether you're in ketosis and how your body is responding to your current carbohydrate intake.

4. Assess Energy Levels and Well-Being: Pay attention to how you feel throughout the day, including your energy levels, mood, and overall well-being. If you experience fatigue, brain fog, or other symptoms of low energy, it may be a sign that you need to adjust your carbohydrate intake.

5. Track Physical Performance: If you engage in regular physical activity or exercise, monitor your performance and recovery. Adjust your carbohydrate intake as needed to support your activity level and ensure adequate energy for workouts.

6. Listen to Hunger and Fullness Signals: Pay attention to your body's hunger and fullness cues. If you're consistently hungry or unsatisfied after meals, it may indicate that you need to adjust your macronutrient ratios, including carbohydrates, to better meet your needs.

7. Consult with a Healthcare Professional: If you're unsure how to adjust your carbohydrate intake or if you're experiencing challenges with ketosis or weight loss, consider consulting with a healthcare professional or registered dietitian who is knowledgeable about the Atkins diet. They can provide personalized guidance and support based on your individual needs and goals.

8. Gradual Adjustments: When making adjustments to your carbohydrate intake, do so gradually to avoid drastic changes that could disrupt ketosis or cause fluctuations in energy levels. Increase or decrease your carbohydrate intake by

small increments (e.g., 5-10 grams per day) and monitor your body's response over time.

9. Keep Track of Non-Scale Victories: While the scale is a useful tool for tracking progress, it's not the only measure of success. Pay attention to non-scale victories such as improvements in energy levels, mood, sleep quality, clothing fit, and measurements of body composition (e.g., waist circumference, body fat percentage).

10. Evaluate Carb Tolerance: Assess your individual carbohydrate tolerance by monitoring how your body responds to different levels of carbohydrate intake. Some individuals may be able to tolerate higher levels of carbohydrates while still maintaining ketosis, while others may need to stay within a stricter carb limit.

11. Experiment with Carb Cycling: Consider incorporating carb cycling into your meal plan, where you alternate between higher and lower carbohydrate days based on your activity level and goals. This approach can help you optimize performance, support muscle growth, and enhance metabolic flexibility while still maintaining ketosis overall.

12. Use a Carb Calculator: Use online tools or resources provided by the Atkins diet program to calculate your daily carbohydrate intake based on your individualized needs and goals. Adjust your carbohydrate intake as needed to align with your desired rate of weight loss or maintenance.

13. Consider Time-Restricted Eating: Experiment with time-restricted eating or intermittent fasting protocols, where you restrict your eating window to a certain

number of hours each day. This approach can help regulate insulin levels, enhance fat burning, and improve metabolic health while still supporting ketosis.

14. Monitor Blood Sugar Levels: If you have diabetes or are concerned about blood sugar control, consider monitoring your blood sugar levels regularly to assess how your carbohydrate intake is affecting your metabolic health. Work with a healthcare professional to interpret your results and make appropriate adjustments to your diet as needed.

15. Stay Educated and Informed: Continuously educate yourself about the principles of the Atkins diet, including the role of carbohydrates, fats, and proteins in ketosis and weight loss. Stay informed about the latest research and recommendations related to low-carb diets to make informed decisions about your dietary choices.

16. Be Patient and Flexible: Remember that achieving and maintaining ketosis is a journey that requires patience, experimentation, and flexibility. Don't be discouraged by temporary setbacks or plateaus, and be open to adjusting your approach based on your evolving needs and goals.

<u>Exercise recommendations for Phase 2</u>

In Phase 2 of the Atkins diet, also known as the "Balancing Phase," incorporating regular physical activity is an important component of achieving and maintaining overall health and weight loss goals. Exercise can enhance metabolic flexibility, support muscle preservation, improve cardiovascular health, and boost mood and energy levels. Here are some exercise recommendations for Phase 2 as an Atkins diet patient:

1. Cardiovascular Exercise: Engage in moderate-intensity cardiovascular exercise most days of the week for at least 30 minutes per session. Activities such as brisk walking, cycling, swimming, dancing, or using cardio machines like ellipticals or treadmills can help burn calories, improve cardiovascular health, and support weight loss.

2. Strength Training: Incorporate strength training exercises into your routine at least two to three times per week. Focus on full-body exercises that target major muscle groups such as squats, lunges, deadlifts, push-ups, rows, and overhead presses. Strength training helps build and preserve lean muscle mass, which is important for metabolic health and overall strength and function.

3. Flexibility and Mobility Work: Don't forget to include flexibility and mobility exercises in your routine to improve joint range of motion, reduce stiffness, and prevent injury. Incorporate activities such as yoga, Pilates, stretching, foam rolling, or mobility drills to enhance flexibility and promote overall physical well-being.

4. Interval Training: Incorporate interval training or high-intensity interval training (HIIT) workouts into your routine to maximize calorie burn, improve cardiovascular fitness, and enhance metabolic efficiency. Alternating between periods of high-intensity exercise and recovery periods can help increase fat burning and improve overall fitness levels.

5. Active Lifestyle: In addition to structured exercise sessions, focus on increasing your overall daily activity levels by incorporating more movement into your daily routine. This can include activities such as taking the stairs instead of the elevator,

parking farther away from your destination, gardening, playing with pets or children, or incorporating more movement breaks throughout the day.

6. Listen to Your Body: Pay attention to your body's signals and adjust your exercise routine accordingly. If you're feeling fatigued or experiencing muscle soreness, consider scaling back the intensity or duration of your workouts and allowing for adequate rest and recovery time.

7. Stay Hydrated and Nourished: Drink plenty of water before, during, and after exercise to stay hydrated and support optimal performance. Fuel your workouts with a balanced meal or snack that includes protein, healthy fats, and carbohydrates to provide sustained energy and support muscle recovery.

8. Consult with a Healthcare Professional: Before starting any new exercise program, especially if you have underlying health conditions or concerns, consult with a healthcare professional or certified fitness trainer who can provide personalized guidance and recommendations based on your individual needs and goals.

9. Progressive Overload: Gradually increase the intensity, duration, or resistance of your workouts over time to continue challenging your body and making progress. This principle of progressive overload is essential for improving fitness levels, building strength, and achieving optimal results.

10. Variety: Incorporate a variety of exercises and activities into your routine to prevent boredom, target different muscle groups, and avoid overuse injuries. Mix

up your workouts with different types of cardio, strength training exercises, and flexibility work to keep your body and mind engaged.

11. Mind-Body Connection: Pay attention to your mind-body connection during exercise by focusing on proper form, breathing, and mindfulness techniques. This can help enhance your workout performance, reduce stress levels, and improve overall well-being.

12. Rest and Recovery: Allow for adequate rest and recovery time between workouts to allow your muscles to repair and rebuild. Incorporate active recovery activities such as gentle stretching, foam rolling, or low-intensity activities like walking or yoga on rest days to promote recovery and reduce muscle soreness.

13. Listen to Your Body: Be mindful of how your body responds to exercise and adjust your routine accordingly. If you experience pain, discomfort, or excessive fatigue, it's important to listen to your body's signals and modify your workouts as needed to prevent injury and support recovery.

14. Set Realistic Goals: Set realistic and achievable fitness goals that align with your overall health and weight loss objectives. Whether it's improving cardiovascular endurance, increasing muscle strength, or reaching a specific fitness milestone, having clear goals can help motivate you to stay consistent with your exercise routine.

15. Accountability and Support: Consider exercising with a workout buddy, joining a fitness class or group, or working with a personal trainer to stay accountable and

motivated. Having support from others can help you stay on track with your exercise goals and make exercise more enjoyable.

16. Enjoyment and Balance: Choose activities and exercises that you enjoy and that fit into your lifestyle. Finding activities that you look forward to can help make exercise a sustainable habit in the long term. Additionally, strive to maintain balance in your exercise routine by incorporating rest days, varying the intensity of your workouts, and prioritizing activities that bring you joy and fulfillment.

Chapter 5: Phase 3: Pre-Maintenance

Gradually increasing carb intake

Gradually increasing carbohydrate intake as an Atkins diet patient during Phase 2 requires a systematic approach to ensure a smooth transition while maintaining ketosis and achieving your health and weight loss goals. Here's how you can gradually increase your carb intake:

1. Monitor Your Progress: Start by monitoring your progress during Phase 1 of the Atkins diet, also known as the Induction Phase. Track your weight loss, energy levels, and overall well-being to establish a baseline for future adjustments.

2. Calculate Your Carb Tolerance: Determine your individual carbohydrate tolerance by gradually increasing your daily carbohydrate intake while monitoring your body's response. Start with an additional 5-10 grams of carbohydrates per day and assess how your body reacts.

3. Choose Low-Glycemic Carbohydrates: Focus on incorporating low-glycemic carbohydrates that have a minimal impact on blood sugar levels and insulin response. Choose whole, unprocessed foods such as non-starchy vegetables, berries, nuts, seeds, and legumes to gradually increase your carb intake.

4. Increase Carbs in Small Increments: Gradually increase your carbohydrate intake by small increments, such as 5-10 grams per week, to allow your body to adapt and maintain ketosis. Monitor your ketone levels, weight, energy levels, and cravings to gauge your body's response.

5. Diversify Your Carb Sources: Incorporate a variety of carbohydrate sources into your meals to ensure a balanced and nutrient-rich diet. Experiment with different types of vegetables, fruits, whole grains, and legumes to increase dietary variety while staying within your carb limit.

6. Monitor Portion Sizes: Pay attention to portion sizes when adding carbohydrates to your meals to avoid overconsumption. Use measuring tools or visual cues to help you accurately portion out carbohydrate-rich foods and stay within your daily carb limit.

7. Adjust Based on Your Goals: Adjust your carbohydrate intake based on your individual health and weight loss goals. If your primary goal is weight loss, you may need to keep your carb intake lower to promote fat burning and maintain ketosis. If your goal is weight maintenance or improved athletic performance, you may be able to tolerate a higher carb intake.

8. Listen to Your Body: Pay attention to how your body responds to the gradual increase in carbohydrate intake. Be mindful of any changes in energy levels, cravings, mood, digestion, or weight fluctuations, and adjust your carb intake accordingly to support your overall well-being.

9. Consult with a Healthcare Professional: If you're unsure how to adjust your carbohydrate intake or if you have underlying health conditions or concerns, consult with a healthcare professional or registered dietitian who is knowledgeable about the Atkins diet. They can provide personalized guidance and support based on your individual needs and goals.

10. Focus on Net Carbs: Pay attention to net carbs, which are calculated by subtracting fiber and certain sugar alcohols from the total carbohydrate content of a food. Net carbs are the carbohydrates that impact blood sugar levels and should be monitored closely on the Atkins diet. Aim to gradually increase your net carb intake while staying within your individualized carb tolerance.

11. Reintroduce Carbohydrates Strategically: When reintroducing carbohydrates into your diet, focus on nutrient-dense, whole food sources that provide essential vitamins, minerals, and fiber. This includes vegetables, fruits, whole grains, and legumes. Start with small portions and gradually increase the amount as your body adapts.

12. Monitor Ketosis: Keep track of your ketone levels using ketone testing strips or a blood ketone meter to ensure that you're staying in ketosis while gradually increasing your carbohydrate intake. This will help you determine your individualized carbohydrate threshold for maintaining ketosis.

13. Be Mindful of Timing: Pay attention to the timing of your carbohydrate intake and how it affects your energy levels and cravings. Some individuals may prefer to consume carbohydrates earlier in the day to provide sustained energy, while others may find it more beneficial to include them in the evening or around workouts.

14. Experiment with Carb Cycling: Consider incorporating carb cycling into your meal plan, where you alternate between higher and lower carb days based on your activity level and goals. This approach can help you strategically increase your carb intake while still supporting ketosis overall.

15. Listen to Your Body's Signals: Pay attention to how your body responds to the gradual increase in carbohydrate intake. Notice any changes in energy levels, mood, digestion, cravings, or weight fluctuations, and adjust your carb intake accordingly to support your overall well-being.

16. Stay Hydrated: Drink plenty of water throughout the day, especially as you increase your carbohydrate intake. Adequate hydration is essential for supporting digestion, metabolism, and overall health, and can help mitigate potential side effects of increasing carbs such as water retention.

17. Track Your Progress: Continue to track your progress by monitoring your weight, measurements, energy levels, mood, and overall well-being. This will help you assess the effectiveness of your carbohydrate intake and make any necessary adjustments to optimize your health and weight loss goals.

By gradually increasing your carbohydrate intake in a controlled manner and paying attention to your body's feedback, you can effectively transition from Phase 1 to Phase 2 of the Atkins diet while optimizing your health and weight loss journey. Remember to be patient, consistent, and mindful of your dietary choices as you make adjustments to your carb intake.

<u>Learning to maintain weight loss</u>

Learning to maintain weight loss as an Atkins diet patient involves adopting sustainable lifestyle habits, making mindful food choices, staying active, and prioritizing overall health and well-being. Here's how you can effectively maintain weight loss while following the Atkins diet:

1. Establish Healthy Eating Patterns: Transition from a restrictive diet mindset to a balanced and sustainable approach to eating. Focus on incorporating a variety of nutrient-dense foods such as lean proteins, healthy fats, non-starchy vegetables, and low-glycemic carbohydrates into your meals. Aim for portion control, mindful eating, and listening to your body's hunger and fullness cues.

2. Monitor Your Carb Intake: Continue to monitor your carbohydrate intake even after reaching your weight loss goals. Find your individualized carbohydrate tolerance level that allows you to maintain your weight without regaining excess pounds. This may require periodic adjustments based on your activity level, metabolic rate, and overall health.

3. Practice Portion Control: Be mindful of portion sizes and avoid overeating, even if you're consuming low-carb foods. Use measuring tools, portion plates, or visual cues to help you gauge appropriate portion sizes and prevent excess calorie intake.

4. Stay Active: Maintain a regular exercise routine that includes a mix of cardiovascular exercise, strength training, flexibility work, and active lifestyle habits. Aim for at least 150 minutes of moderate-intensity aerobic activity or 75 minutes of vigorous-intensity activity per week, along with muscle-strengthening activities on two or more days per week.

5. Prioritize Protein and Fiber: Continue to prioritize protein-rich foods and fiber-rich carbohydrates in your meals to support satiety, muscle maintenance, and digestive health. Lean proteins, such as poultry, fish, tofu, and legumes, can help keep you feeling full and satisfied, while fiber-rich vegetables, fruits, and whole grains can help regulate blood sugar levels and promote digestive regularity.

6. Stay Hydrated: Drink plenty of water throughout the day to stay hydrated and support overall health. Adequate hydration can help prevent overeating, support metabolism, and promote optimal body function. Aim for at least eight glasses of water per day, or more if you're physically active or in a hot climate.

7. Practice Mindful Eating: Be mindful of your eating habits and make conscious choices about what, when, and how much you eat. Avoid mindless snacking, emotional eating, and eating out of boredom. Pay attention to your body's hunger and fullness cues, and eat slowly to savor your food and prevent overeating.

8. Monitor Your Progress: Continue to monitor your weight, measurements, energy levels, mood, and overall well-being regularly to track your progress and make any necessary adjustments to your lifestyle habits. Celebrate your achievements and be proactive in addressing any challenges or setbacks that may arise.

9. Seek Support and Accountability: Surround yourself with a supportive network of friends, family, or a weight loss maintenance group who can provide encouragement, motivation, and accountability as you work to maintain your weight loss. Share your successes, challenges, and goals with others who understand and support your journey.

10. Focus on Long-Term Health: Shift your focus from short-term weight loss goals to long-term health and well-being. Embrace the Atkins diet as a sustainable lifestyle that promotes overall health, vitality, and longevity. Make self-care a priority, practice stress management techniques, get adequate sleep, and prioritize mental and emotional well-being.

11. Regular Self-Monitoring: Continue to track your food intake, physical activity, and weight regularly to stay accountable and aware of your progress. Self-monitoring can help you identify any patterns or behaviors that may be affecting your weight and make adjustments as needed.

12. Plan and Prepare Meals: Plan your meals and snacks in advance to avoid impulsive food choices and overeating. Stock your kitchen with healthy, Atkins-friendly foods and ingredients, and prepare meals in batches to make healthy eating convenient and accessible throughout the week.

13. Incorporate Indulgence Wisely: While the Atkins diet emphasizes low-carb, nutrient-dense foods, there is still room for occasional indulgences. Allow yourself to enjoy treats or higher-carb foods in moderation, but be mindful of portion sizes and frequency to prevent derailing your progress.

14. Focus on Sustainable Habits: Shift your focus from short-term dieting to long-term lifestyle habits that support weight maintenance and overall health. Embrace a balanced approach to eating that includes a variety of nutrient-dense foods, regular physical activity, adequate sleep, stress management, and self-care practices.

15. Stay Educated: Continue to educate yourself about nutrition, health, and wellness to make informed choices that support your weight maintenance goals. Stay up-to-date on the latest research, trends, and recommendations related to low-carb diets, and seek out reputable sources of information and support.

16. Find Balance: Strive for balance in your eating habits and lifestyle. Allow yourself to enjoy occasional indulgences and social events without guilt, but also prioritize nourishing your body with healthy, whole foods and engaging in regular physical activity to maintain your overall well-being.

17. Celebrate Non-Scale Victories: Celebrate your successes and achievements beyond the number on the scale. Focus on non-scale victories such as improvements in energy levels, mood, confidence, physical fitness, and overall quality of life as indicators of your progress and success.

18. Be Kind to Yourself: Be patient and compassionate with yourself as you navigate the ups and downs of weight maintenance. Recognize that maintaining weight loss is a lifelong journey that may have its challenges, and be gentle with yourself during times of struggle or setbacks.

19. Stay Connected: Stay connected with your support network of friends, family, or online communities who can provide encouragement, motivation, and accountability as you work to maintain your weight loss. Share your experiences, challenges, and successes with others who understand and support your journey.

20. Adapt and Adjust: Be open to adapting and adjusting your approach as needed to support your evolving needs and goals. Listen to your body, be flexible with your eating and exercise routines, and be willing to make changes that promote your long-term health and well-being.

<u>Strategies for overcoming plateaus</u>

Overcoming plateaus as an Atkins diet patient can be challenging, but with the right strategies, you can break through barriers and continue making progress towards your weight loss and health goals. Here are some effective strategies for overcoming plateaus on the Atkins diet:

1. Review Your Eating Habits: Take a closer look at your eating habits and food choices to identify any areas where you may be slipping or overindulging. Are you accurately tracking your carbohydrate intake? Are you consuming hidden sources of carbs or processed foods? Assessing your eating habits can help pinpoint areas for improvement.

2. Reassess Your Carbohydrate Intake: If you've been following the same carbohydrate intake for a while, it may be time to reassess and potentially adjust your carb intake. Gradually reduce your carb intake by 5-10 grams per day to kickstart fat burning and stimulate weight loss. Experiment with different levels of carb restriction to find what works best for your body.

3. Increase Protein Intake: Protein is essential for muscle maintenance and satiety, so increasing your protein intake can help boost metabolism and curb cravings. Incorporate protein-rich foods such as lean meats, poultry, fish, eggs, tofu, and legumes into your meals to support weight loss and overcome plateaus.

4. Incorporate Intermittent Fasting: Intermittent fasting can help break through weight loss plateaus by promoting fat burning and improving metabolic flexibility. Experiment with different fasting protocols, such as 16/8, where you fast for 16 hours and eat within an 8-hour window, to see if it helps jumpstart your progress.

5. Vary Your Exercise Routine: If you've hit a plateau in your weight loss journey, it may be time to shake up your exercise routine. Incorporate new forms of

exercise, increase the intensity or duration of your workouts, or try different types of activities such as interval training, strength training, or high-intensity interval training (HIIT) to challenge your body and stimulate fat loss.

6. Prioritize Sleep and Stress Management: Poor sleep and high stress levels can negatively impact weight loss efforts and contribute to plateaus. Prioritize quality sleep and stress management techniques such as meditation, yoga, deep breathing exercises, or mindfulness practices to support overall well-being and optimize weight loss.

7. Stay Hydrated: Adequate hydration is essential for metabolism, digestion, and overall health. Drink plenty of water throughout the day to stay hydrated and support weight loss. Sometimes, dehydration can mask itself as a weight loss plateau, so ensure you're drinking enough water daily.

8. Be Patient and Persistent: Plateaus are a normal part of the weight loss journey, and it's important to stay patient and persistent during these times. Trust the process, stay committed to your goals, and continue making healthy choices even when progress seems slow. Remember that weight loss is not always linear, and consistency is key to long-term success.

9. Seek Support and Accountability: Surround yourself with a supportive network of friends, family, or fellow Atkins dieters who can provide encouragement, motivation, and accountability during plateaus. Share your experiences, challenges, and successes with others who understand and support your journey.

10. Consult with a Healthcare Professional: If you're struggling to overcome a weight loss plateau despite your best efforts, consider consulting with a healthcare professional or registered dietitian who is knowledgeable about the Atkins diet. They can provide personalized guidance, support, and recommendations based on your individual needs and goals.

11. Periodic Carb Cycling: Experiment with carb cycling, where you alternate between higher and lower carb days. This can help prevent metabolic adaptation and keep your body responsive to changes. On higher carb days, focus on healthy, nutrient-dense carbs like sweet potatoes, quinoa, or fruits.

12. Track Non-Scale Progress: Don't solely rely on the scale for progress. Monitor other indicators such as changes in body measurements, clothing fit, increased energy levels, improved mood, and enhanced physical performance. These non-scale victories can be valuable indicators of success.

13. Review Hidden Carbs and Ingredients: Reassess your food choices for hidden carbs and ingredients that might be impacting your progress. Processed foods, sauces, and condiments can sometimes contain hidden sugars or starches. Check labels carefully to ensure you're staying within your carb limits.

14. Consider Thermic Effect of Food (TEF): Understand the concept of the thermic effect of food – the energy expended during digestion. Protein has a higher TEF compared to fats and carbs, meaning your body burns more calories digesting protein. Consider adjusting your macronutrient ratios to include more protein.

15. Dial-In Your Macros: Reevaluate your macronutrient ratios. Adjusting the balance of fats, proteins, and carbs may help kickstart your metabolism. Increasing healthy fats while moderating protein and carb intake can be a strategic approach, but individual responses vary.

16. Implement Refeeds: Introduce occasional refeed days where you deliberately increase your carb intake. This can help prevent metabolic adaptation and give your body a temporary boost in leptin, a hormone involved in regulating energy expenditure.

17. Stay Consistent with Exercise: Consistency is key when it comes to exercise. Ensure you're maintaining a regular workout routine that includes a mix of cardiovascular exercise and strength training. Increasing muscle mass can positively impact your metabolism.

18. Modify Intensity and Duration of Workouts: If your exercise routine has become routine, shake things up. Increase the intensity or duration of your workouts to challenge your body. Consider incorporating high-intensity interval training (HIIT) or adding resistance to your strength training routine.

19. Evaluate Hormonal Factors: Hormones play a crucial role in weight management. Factors like stress, sleep, and hormonal fluctuations can impact weight loss. Prioritize stress management techniques, get adequate sleep, and consider consulting with a healthcare professional if you suspect hormonal imbalances.

20. Set Realistic Expectations: Plateaus are a normal part of any weight loss journey. Set realistic expectations and understand that weight loss may not always be linear. Focus on creating sustainable habits and celebrate the progress you've made.

21. Consider Time-Restricted Eating: Experiment with time-restricted eating or intermittent fasting. This approach involves restricting your eating window, potentially helping to regulate insulin levels and promote fat burning. However, it's essential to find a pattern that fits your lifestyle.

22. Reevaluate Snacking Habits: While snacking can be part of a healthy diet, reassess your snacking habits. Mindless snacking or grazing throughout the day might contribute to hidden calorie intake. Opt for nutrient-dense snacks and be mindful of portion sizes.

<u>Balancing macronutrients for long-term success</u>

Balancing macronutrients for long-term success as an Atkins diet patient is essential for achieving optimal health, sustained weight loss, and overall well-being. The Atkins diet focuses on controlling carbohydrate intake while emphasizing adequate protein and healthy fats. Here are some key principles and strategies for balancing macronutrients on the Atkins diet for long-term success:

1. Prioritize Protein: Protein is a crucial macronutrient that supports muscle maintenance, satiety, and metabolic health. Aim to include a source of protein in each meal and snack to help control hunger, stabilize blood sugar levels, and preserve lean muscle mass. Good sources of protein on the Atkins diet include poultry, fish, eggs, tofu, tempeh, legumes, and low-carb protein powders.

2. Moderate Carbohydrate Intake: Control your carbohydrate intake by focusing on low-glycemic, nutrient-dense carbohydrates that have a minimal impact on blood sugar levels. Non-starchy vegetables, leafy greens, berries, nuts, seeds, and small portions of whole grains are excellent choices. Limit or avoid high-carb foods such as refined grains, sugars, starchy vegetables, and processed snacks.

3. Include Healthy Fats: Healthy fats are an essential component of the Atkins diet and provide a concentrated source of energy, support hormone production, and aid in nutrient absorption. Include a variety of healthy fats in your meals, such as avocados, olive oil, nuts, seeds, fatty fish, and coconut oil. Aim for a balance of monounsaturated, polyunsaturated, and saturated fats to support overall health.

4. Calculate Macronutrient Ratios: Determine your personalized macronutrient ratios based on your individual needs, goals, and preferences. While the Atkins diet generally emphasizes higher fat intake and moderate protein intake with low-carb foods, the specific ratios may vary depending on factors such as activity level, metabolic rate, and weight loss goals.

5. Adjust Based on Progress: Monitor your progress and adjust your macronutrient intake as needed to support your long-term goals. If you're not seeing the desired results, consider tweaking your macronutrient ratios by adjusting your protein, fat, and carbohydrate intake accordingly. Experiment with different ratios to find what works best for your body.

6. Listen to Your Body: Pay attention to your body's hunger and fullness cues, energy levels, mood, and overall well-being to guide your macronutrient choices.

Everyone's nutritional needs are unique, so it's essential to listen to your body and make adjustments based on how you feel.

7. Stay Hydrated: Adequate hydration is crucial for optimal health and weight management. Drink plenty of water throughout the day to stay hydrated and support digestion, metabolism, and overall well-being. Consider adding electrolytes or mineral-rich beverages to your routine, especially if you're following a low-carb diet.

8. Plan Balanced Meals: Create balanced meals that include a combination of protein, healthy fats, and low-carb vegetables or fruits. Aim for variety and color on your plate to ensure you're getting a wide range of nutrients and phytonutrients. Experiment with different recipes and meal combinations to keep your meals exciting and satisfying.

9. Prioritize Whole Foods: Choose whole, minimally processed foods whenever possible to maximize nutrient intake and support overall health. Whole foods provide essential vitamins, minerals, antioxidants, and fiber that are essential for optimal health and well-being. Limit or avoid processed foods, artificial ingredients, and additives that can detract from your long-term success.

10. Be Patient and Consistent: Achieving and maintaining macronutrient balance takes time, patience, and consistency. Focus on making gradual, sustainable changes to your eating habits and lifestyle, and trust the process. Celebrate your progress and stay committed to your long-term health and well-being.

11. Track Your Macronutrients: Use a food tracking app or journal to track your daily intake of macronutrients (carbohydrates, protein, and fat). This can help you gain a better understanding of your eating habits and ensure you're meeting your macronutrient goals.

12. Focus on Quality: While macronutrient balance is important, prioritize the quality of your food choices. Choose whole, nutrient-dense foods that provide essential vitamins, minerals, and antioxidants. Opt for organic, grass-fed, and pasture-raised options whenever possible to maximize nutrient content and support overall health.

13. Mindful Eating: Practice mindful eating by paying attention to your hunger and fullness cues, as well as the taste, texture, and enjoyment of your food. Avoid distractions while eating, such as watching TV or scrolling on your phone, and take the time to savor and appreciate your meals.

14. Adjust Portions: Pay attention to portion sizes to ensure you're not overeating or under-eating certain macronutrients. Use measuring cups, food scales, or visual cues to help you portion out appropriate serving sizes of protein, fats, and carbohydrates.

15. Experiment with Intermittent Fasting: Consider incorporating intermittent fasting into your routine, which involves cycling between periods of eating and fasting. This can help regulate appetite, improve insulin sensitivity, and promote fat loss while still allowing you to maintain balanced macronutrient intake.

16. Listen to Your Body: Your body's needs may change over time, so be open to adjusting your macronutrient intake based on how you feel. Pay attention to any changes in energy levels, mood, digestion, or weight fluctuations, and adjust your macronutrient ratios accordingly.

17. Stay Consistent: Consistency is key when it comes to balancing macronutrients for long-term success. Stick to your meal plan and make healthy choices consistently, even on weekends or during special occasions. This can help prevent fluctuations in macronutrient intake and support sustained progress towards your goals.

18. Seek Professional Guidance: If you're struggling to balance your macronutrients or have specific dietary concerns, consider consulting with a registered dietitian or nutritionist who specializes in the Atkins diet or low-carb nutrition. They can provide personalized guidance, support, and recommendations based on your individual needs and goals.

19. Be Flexible: While it's important to have a general framework for balancing macronutrients, be flexible and adaptable with your approach. Your dietary needs may vary depending on factors such as activity level, metabolic rate, and health status. Don't be afraid to experiment with different macronutrient ratios to find what works best for you.

20. Celebrate Progress: Celebrate your progress and achievements along the way. Recognize the positive changes you've made in your eating habits and lifestyle, and acknowledge the hard work and dedication you've put into balancing your macronutrients for long-term success.

Chapter 6: Phase 4: Lifetime Maintenance

Establishing a sustainable eating pattern

Establishing a sustainable eating pattern as an Atkins diet patient involves focusing on whole, nutrient-dense foods while limiting processed and refined carbohydrates. This includes incorporating plenty of vegetables, lean proteins, healthy fats, and low-carb fruits into your meals. It's important to listen to your body's hunger and fullness cues, and to stay hydrated. Regular physical activity and meal planning can also support long-term success on the Atkins diet.

Here are some tips for establishing a sustainable eating pattern while following the Atkins diet:

1. Focus on Whole Foods: Emphasize whole, minimally processed foods such as vegetables, fruits, nuts, seeds, lean proteins (e.g., poultry, fish, tofu), and healthy fats (e.g., avocados, olive oil, nuts).

2. Limit Processed Carbohydrates: Minimize intake of processed and refined carbohydrates such as white bread, pasta, sugary snacks, and sugary beverages. Instead, opt for high-fiber, low-carb alternatives like whole grains, legumes, and low-carb sweeteners (if needed).

3. Monitor Carb Intake: Pay attention to your carbohydrate intake and aim to stay within your recommended carb allowance for your specific phase of the Atkins diet. This may involve tracking carb grams or using the Atkins app to help monitor your daily intake.

4. Stay Hydrated: Drink plenty of water throughout the day to stay hydrated, support digestion, and help control appetite. Herbal teas and sugar-free beverages can also be included, but be cautious of hidden sugars in some beverages.

5. Include Non-Starchy Vegetables: Non-starchy vegetables such as leafy greens, broccoli, cauliflower, peppers, and zucchini are low in carbohydrates and rich in vitamins, minerals, and fiber. Aim to include a variety of colorful vegetables in your meals for optimal nutrition.

6. Choose Healthy Fats: Incorporate sources of healthy fats into your meals, such as avocados, nuts, seeds, olive oil, and fatty fish like salmon. These fats provide essential nutrients and can help keep you feeling satisfied between meals.

7. Plan and Prep Meals: Planning and preparing meals ahead of time can help you stay on track with your eating plan. Batch cooking, meal prepping, and having healthy snacks readily available can prevent impulsive food choices and make it easier to stick to your dietary goals.

8. Listen to Your Body: Pay attention to your body's hunger and fullness cues, and eat mindfully. Avoid skipping meals or waiting until you're overly hungry, as this can lead to overeating or making less healthy food choices.

9. Regular Physical Activity: Incorporate regular physical activity into your routine to support overall health and weight management. Choose activities you enjoy, whether it's walking, cycling, swimming, or yoga, and aim for at least 150 minutes of moderate-intensity exercise per week.

10. Seek Support and Guidance: Consider working with a registered dietitian or healthcare provider who is knowledgeable about the Atkins diet to receive personalized guidance, support, and encouragement on your journey toward establishing a sustainable eating pattern.

Certainly! Here are some additional insights and considerations for establishing a sustainable eating pattern as an Atkins diet patient:

11. Mindful Eating: Practice mindful eating by paying attention to the taste, texture, and satisfaction level of your food. Eating slowly and savoring each bite can help prevent overeating and enhance your enjoyment of meals.

12. Variety and Balance: Aim for variety in your food choices to ensure you're getting a wide range of nutrients. Include a mix of different proteins, vegetables, fats, and low-carb fruits to promote nutritional balance and prevent boredom with your meals.

13. Social Support: Surround yourself with supportive friends, family members, or online communities who understand and respect your dietary choices. Having a support system can make it easier to navigate social situations and stay committed to your eating plan.

14. Flexibility: While the Atkins diet provides guidelines for carbohydrate intake, it's important to be flexible and adjust your eating plan based on your individual needs, preferences, and lifestyle. Allow yourself occasional treats or higher-carb meals while staying mindful of portion sizes and overall balance.

15. Monitor Progress: Keep track of your progress on the Atkins diet by monitoring factors such as weight, energy levels, mood, and overall well-being. Regularly reassess your goals and make adjustments to your eating plan as needed to ensure continued success.

16. Education and Resources: Take advantage of resources such as cookbooks, meal plans, online forums, and educational materials provided by Atkins or other reputable sources. Continuing to learn about low-carb eating and staying informed about new research can help you make informed choices and stay motivated.

17. Addressing Challenges: Be prepared to face challenges and setbacks along the way, such as cravings, social pressures, or plateaus in weight loss. Develop strategies for coping with these challenges, such as finding healthier alternatives to high-carb foods, practicing stress management techniques, or seeking professional support if needed.

18. Long-Term Maintenance: As you progress on the Atkins diet and reach your desired weight or health goals, shift your focus toward long-term maintenance. This may involve gradually increasing your carbohydrate intake while continuing to prioritize whole, nutrient-dense foods and mindful eating habits.

19. Celebrate Success: Celebrate your achievements and milestones on the Atkins diet, whether it's reaching a weight loss goal, improving your health markers, or mastering new cooking skills. Acknowledge your progress and recognize the positive changes you've made in your lifestyle.

20. Lifestyle Integration: Finally, strive to integrate the principles of the Atkins diet into your overall lifestyle for sustainable health and well-being. Embrace a balanced approach to eating, exercise, stress management, and self-care that supports your long-term goals and enhances your quality of life.

<u>Managing social situations and dining out</u>

Managing social situations and dining out can present challenges for individuals following the Atkins diet, but with some planning and flexibility, it's entirely manageable. Here's a guide to help navigate these situations effectively:

1. Plan Ahead: Before attending social events or dining out, review the menu options if possible. Many restaurants now provide online menus with nutritional information, which can help you make informed choices in advance.

2. Communicate Your Needs: Don't be afraid to communicate your dietary preferences and needs to the host or restaurant staff. Most establishments are willing to accommodate special requests or modifications to dishes.

3. Focus on Protein and Vegetables: When dining out, look for options that center around protein and non-starchy vegetables. This might include grilled meats, seafood, salads, and vegetable sides. Ask for dressings and sauces on the side to control the amount of added sugars or carbs.

4. Substitute Smartly: Be creative with substitutions to lower the carb content of your meal. For example, swap out high-carb sides like potatoes or rice for extra vegetables or a side salad. Requesting steamed or sautéed vegetables instead of bread or pasta can also reduce carb intake.

5. Beware of Hidden Carbs: Be mindful of hidden sources of carbohydrates in sauces, marinades, and dressings. Opt for options that are grilled, baked, or broiled rather than breaded or fried, as breading can add unnecessary carbs.

6. Portion Control: Pay attention to portion sizes, especially when dining out where portions tend to be larger than what you might typically eat at home. Consider sharing entrees or asking for a to-go box to save half for another meal.

7. Stay Hydrated: Drink water or other non-caloric beverages throughout the meal to stay hydrated and help control appetite. Avoid sugary drinks and excessive alcohol, which can add unnecessary carbs and calories.

8. Be Flexible: While it's essential to stick to your dietary goals, it's also important to be flexible and enjoy social occasions without feeling deprived. If you indulge in a higher-carb meal or dessert occasionally, focus on getting back on track with your eating plan the next day.

9. Bring Your Own Dish: If you're attending a potluck or gathering where food options may be limited, consider bringing a dish that aligns with your dietary preferences. This ensures that you have at least one option that you can enjoy guilt-free.

10. Focus on Socializing: Remember that social occasions are about more than just food. Focus on enjoying the company of friends and family, and don't let dietary concerns overshadow the social aspect of the event.

11. Anticipate Challenges: Be prepared for potential challenges and temptations that may arise in social situations or at restaurants. Visualize how you will handle these situations beforehand and have a plan in place to stay on track with your dietary goals.

12. Choose Wisely: When faced with a buffet or a wide array of food options, take your time to carefully choose the foods that align with your dietary preferences. Focus on filling your plate with protein-rich foods, salads, and vegetables, and be mindful of portion sizes.

13. Customize Your Order: Don't hesitate to customize your order at restaurants to meet your dietary needs. Ask for substitutions, modifications, or special requests to create a meal that fits within the Atkins guidelines. Most restaurants are willing to accommodate dietary preferences, so don't be afraid to ask.

14. Be Assertive: Be assertive when communicating your dietary needs to restaurant staff or hosts. Clearly communicate any allergies, intolerances, or dietary restrictions, and don't feel obligated to eat foods that don't align with your goals.

15. Seek Support: If you're attending a social event where food will be served, consider bringing a supportive friend or family member who understands your dietary preferences. Having someone who can offer encouragement and support can make it easier to stick to your eating plan.

16. Practice Moderation: If you're faced with a tempting dessert or high-carb dish, practice moderation by enjoying a small portion instead of completely avoiding it. Savor each bite mindfully and focus on quality over quantity.

17. Stay Mindful: Stay mindful of your hunger and fullness cues throughout the meal. Avoid mindless snacking or overeating out of boredom or social pressure. Take breaks between bites, sip water, and engage in conversation to pace yourself.

18. Be Flexible: While it's important to stick to the principles of the Atkins diet, it's also essential to be flexible and adaptable in social situations. Remember that occasional deviations from your eating plan are normal and can be managed without derailing your progress.

19. Prepare for Success: Set yourself up for success by planning ahead for social events and dining out. Bring low-carb snacks or emergency food options in case healthy choices are limited. Having backup options on hand can help prevent impulsive food choices.

20. Celebrate Non-Food Activities: Shift the focus of social gatherings away from food by incorporating non-food activities such as games, walks, or other shared experiences. This can help reduce the emphasis on food and make it easier to stick to your dietary goals.

Certainly! Here are some further insights and tips for managing social situations and dining out while following the Atkins diet:

21. Research Restaurant Options: Before dining out, research restaurants in your area that offer low-carb or keto-friendly options. Many restaurants now cater to various dietary preferences and may have specific menu items or modifications that align with the Atkins diet.

22. Ask Questions: Don't hesitate to ask questions about menu items, ingredients, and preparation methods when dining out. Restaurant staff can provide valuable information to help you make informed choices that fit within your dietary goals.

23. Look for Hidden Carbs: Be mindful of hidden sources of carbohydrates in restaurant meals, such as breaded meats, sauces thickened with flour or sugar, and high-carb sides like mashed potatoes or fries. Ask about ingredient substitutions or modifications to reduce the carb content of your meal.

24. Choose Low-Carb Beverages: Opt for low-carb beverage options such as water, unsweetened tea, coffee, or sparkling water with a splash of lemon or lime. Avoid sugary cocktails, sodas, and other high-carb drinks that can derail your progress on the Atkins diet.

25. Navigate Buffets Wisely: When faced with a buffet, start by surveying all the options before filling your plate. Choose protein-rich dishes like grilled chicken, seafood, or roasted meats, along with plenty of non-starchy vegetables. Avoid or limit high-carb items like bread, pasta, and desserts.

26. Be Prepared for Peer Pressure: Be prepared to face peer pressure or social stigma regarding your dietary choices, especially if they deviate from the norm. Stay confident in your decision to follow the Atkins diet and politely decline offers of foods that don't align with your goals.

27. Bring Your Own Snacks: If you're unsure about the availability of low-carb options at a social gathering or event, consider bringing your own snacks or dishes

to share. This ensures that you have something to eat that fits within your dietary preferences while still participating in the festivities.

28. Practice Mindful Indulgence: If you choose to indulge in higher-carb foods or desserts during special occasions, do so mindfully and without guilt. Enjoy the experience fully, savoring each bite, and return to your regular eating plan afterward without dwelling on any perceived "slip-ups."

29. Find Supportive Friends and Family: Surround yourself with friends and family members who support your dietary choices and understand your commitment to the Atkins diet. Having a supportive network can make it easier to navigate social situations and stay on track with your goals.

30. Stay Positive and Flexible: Remember that the Atkins diet is meant to be a sustainable lifestyle change, not a restrictive diet. Stay positive, flexible, and open-minded as you navigate social situations and dining out, and focus on making choices that support your long-term health and well-being.

<u>Incorporating physical activity for overall health</u>

Incorporating physical activity into your routine is essential for overall health and well-being, especially when following the Atkins diet. Here are some tips on how you can incorporate physical activity into your lifestyle:

1. Choose Activities You Enjoy: Find physical activities that you enjoy and look forward to doing. Whether it's walking, jogging, swimming, cycling, dancing, or playing a sport, choosing activities that you find enjoyable increases the likelihood that you'll stick with them long-term.

2. Set Realistic Goals: Set realistic and achievable goals for physical activity based on your current fitness level and schedule. Start with small, manageable goals and gradually increase the intensity, duration, and frequency of your workouts as you progress.

3. Schedule Regular Exercise Sessions: Treat exercise like any other important appointment and schedule regular workout sessions into your calendar. Consistency is key to seeing results, so aim for at least 150 minutes of moderate-intensity aerobic activity or 75 minutes of vigorous-intensity activity per week, as recommended by health guidelines.

4. Incorporate Strength Training: In addition to cardiovascular exercise, incorporate strength training into your routine to build muscle, improve metabolism, and enhance overall body composition. Bodyweight exercises, resistance bands, free weights, or weight machines can all be effective for strength training.

5. Be Active Throughout the Day: Look for opportunities to be active throughout the day, even if you don't have time for a formal workout. Take the stairs instead of the elevator, park farther away from your destination, or take short breaks to stretch and move around during the day.

6. Mix It Up: Keep your workouts interesting and challenging by varying your routine. Try different types of exercises, switch up your workout environment, or participate in group fitness classes to keep things fun and engaging.

7. Listen to Your Body: Pay attention to your body's cues and adjust your workouts accordingly. If you're feeling fatigued or sore, take a rest day or engage in gentle activities like yoga or stretching to promote recovery.

8. Stay Hydrated: Drink plenty of water before, during, and after exercise to stay hydrated and support optimal performance. Dehydration can impair exercise performance and recovery, so make hydration a priority.

9. Fuel Your Workouts: Eat a balanced meal or snack containing protein and carbohydrates before and after your workouts to fuel your body and support muscle recovery. Experiment with different pre- and post-workout snacks to find what works best for you.

10. Track Your Progress: Keep track of your physical activity and progress over time to stay motivated and accountable. Use a fitness tracker, smartphone app, or journal to log your workouts, track your steps, and monitor your improvements in strength, endurance, and overall fitness.

Of course! Here are some additional tips and considerations for incorporating physical activity into your routine as an Atkins diet patient:

11. Find Accountability: Partnering with a workout buddy, joining a fitness class, or hiring a personal trainer can provide accountability and motivation to stick with your exercise routine. Having someone to support and encourage you can make it easier to stay committed to your fitness goals.

12. Set Specific Goals: Set specific, measurable, and achievable fitness goals to work towards. Whether it's improving endurance, increasing strength, or

completing a specific workout challenge, having clear goals can help keep you focused and motivated.

13. Gradually Increase Intensity: If you're new to exercise or returning after a break, start slowly and gradually increase the intensity and duration of your workouts over time. Listen to your body and avoid pushing yourself too hard, especially in the beginning.

14. Include Flexibility and Mobility Work: Incorporate flexibility and mobility exercises into your routine to improve range of motion, prevent injury, and enhance overall functional fitness. Activities like yoga, Pilates, or stretching routines can help improve flexibility and reduce muscle stiffness.

15. Prioritize Recovery: Allow your body time to rest and recover between workouts. Incorporate rest days into your schedule to prevent burnout and reduce the risk of overtraining. Use techniques like foam rolling, massage, and adequate sleep to support recovery and muscle repair.

16. Be Consistent: Consistency is key when it comes to physical activity. Aim to exercise on a regular basis, ideally incorporating some form of movement into your daily routine. Even small bouts of activity throughout the day can add up and contribute to your overall fitness.

17. Listen to Your Body: Pay attention to how your body responds to different types of exercise and adjust your routine accordingly. If you experience pain or discomfort during a workout, modify the activity or seek guidance from a fitness professional to ensure you're exercising safely and effectively.

18. Stay Motivated: Find ways to stay motivated and engaged with your fitness routine. This could include setting rewards for reaching milestones, tracking your progress visually, or participating in fitness challenges or events.

19. Make It Enjoyable: Choose activities that you genuinely enjoy and look forward to doing. Whether it's dancing, hiking, gardening, or playing a sport, finding activities that bring you joy will make it easier to stick with your exercise routine in the long run.

20. Celebrate Your Achievements: Celebrate your achievements and progress along the way. Whether it's reaching a fitness milestone, mastering a new exercise, or simply being consistent with your workouts, take time to acknowledge and celebrate your accomplishments.

<u>Tips for preventing weight regain</u>

Preventing weight regain is a common concern for individuals following any diet plan, including the Atkins diet. Here are some tips specifically tailored for Atkins diet patients to help prevent weight regain:

1. Stick to Your Carbohydrate Tolerance: Pay close attention to your individual carbohydrate tolerance and aim to stay within the recommended carb intake for your specific phase of the Atkins diet. This helps prevent excessive carb consumption, which can lead to weight regain.

2. Focus on Whole Foods: Emphasize whole, nutrient-dense foods such as vegetables, lean proteins, healthy fats, and low-carb fruits in your diet. These foods

provide essential nutrients and help keep you feeling satisfied, reducing the likelihood of overeating and weight regain.

3. Practice Portion Control: Be mindful of portion sizes, even when eating low-carb foods. Overeating, even on low-carb foods, can still lead to an excess of calories and hinder weight maintenance. Use smaller plates, measure portions, and pay attention to your body's hunger and fullness cues.

4. Monitor Your Intake: Stay vigilant about monitoring your food intake, especially as you transition to different phases of the Atkins diet. Keep track of your carb intake, as well as your overall calorie consumption, to ensure you're staying on track with your weight maintenance goals.

5. Incorporate Physical Activity: Regular physical activity is crucial for weight maintenance and overall health. Aim for a combination of cardiovascular exercise, strength training, and flexibility exercises to support your metabolism, muscle mass, and overall fitness level.

6. Be Mindful of High-Carb Foods: While the Atkins diet allows for some flexibility in carb intake, be cautious of reintroducing high-carb foods too quickly or in large quantities. These foods can easily lead to overconsumption of calories and hinder your weight maintenance efforts.

7. Plan and Prepare Meals: Take the time to plan and prepare your meals in advance to ensure they align with your dietary goals. Batch cooking, meal prepping, and having healthy snacks readily available can help prevent impulsive food choices and support weight maintenance.

8. Stay Hydrated: Drink plenty of water throughout the day to stay hydrated and support your metabolism. Sometimes thirst can be mistaken for hunger, leading to overeating. Aim to drink at least 8 glasses of water per day, or more if you're physically active.

9. Manage Stress: Stress can contribute to weight gain and make it challenging to maintain healthy eating habits. Practice stress-reducing techniques such as meditation, deep breathing, yoga, or engaging in hobbies to help manage stress levels and prevent emotional eating.

10. Seek Support: Don't hesitate to seek support from a registered dietitian, healthcare provider, or support group if you're struggling to maintain your weight on the Atkins diet. They can provide personalized guidance, support, and encouragement to help you stay on track with your weight maintenance goals.
Certainly! Here are some additional tips and strategies for preventing weight regain as an Atkins diet patient:

11. Stay Consistent with Phases: Follow the phases of the Atkins diet as outlined in the program guidelines. Each phase serves a specific purpose in gradually reintroducing carbohydrates while maintaining weight loss. Resist the temptation to skip phases or rush through them, as this can disrupt your body's ability to adapt to changes in carb intake and increase the risk of weight regain.

12. Be Mindful of Alcohol Intake: Alcohol contains calories and can stimulate appetite, making it easier to overeat and potentially regain weight. Be mindful of your alcohol consumption and choose low-carb options like dry wine, spirits, or

light beer in moderation. Avoid sugary cocktails and mixed drinks that are high in carbs.

13. Practice Mindful Eating: Slow down and pay attention to your eating habits. Practice mindful eating by savoring each bite, chewing slowly, and tuning in to your body's hunger and fullness signals. Avoid distractions like screens or eating on the go, which can lead to overeating and weight regain.

14. Stay Active Outside of Formal Exercise: Incorporate physical activity into your daily routine beyond structured workouts. Take the stairs instead of the elevator, walk or bike for short errands, and find opportunities to move throughout the day. Increasing your overall activity level can help prevent weight regain and support long-term weight maintenance.

15. Monitor Your Progress: Regularly assess your progress and make adjustments as needed to prevent weight regain. Use tools like a food diary, weight tracker, or measurements to monitor changes in your body composition and adjust your eating and exercise habits accordingly.

16. Manage Cravings and Temptations: Develop strategies for managing cravings and temptations for high-carb foods. Keep low-carb snacks on hand for moments of hunger or cravings, practice distraction techniques like going for a walk or engaging in a hobby, and focus on the long-term benefits of sticking to your dietary goals.

17. Prioritize Sleep: Aim for adequate sleep each night, as poor sleep quality and insufficient sleep can disrupt hormones that regulate appetite and metabolism,

leading to weight gain. Create a relaxing bedtime routine, avoid caffeine and screens before bed, and strive for 7-9 hours of quality sleep per night.

18. Practice Self-Compassion: Be kind to yourself and practice self-compassion on your weight maintenance journey. Accept that there may be occasional setbacks or fluctuations in weight, and focus on making sustainable lifestyle changes rather than striving for perfection. Celebrate your progress and achievements along the way.

19. Stay Educated: Continue to educate yourself about nutrition, physical activity, and healthy lifestyle habits to support your weight maintenance efforts. Stay informed about updates to the Atkins diet program, research on low-carb eating, and evidence-based strategies for weight management.

20. Seek Professional Support: If you're struggling to prevent weight regain or have concerns about your progress, consider seeking support from a registered dietitian, nutritionist, or healthcare provider who specializes in weight management. They can provide personalized guidance, accountability, and support to help you achieve your goals.

Chapter 7 : Understanding Carbohydrates

Differentiating between good and bad carbs

As an Atkins diet patient, differentiating between good and bad carbs is essential for effectively managing your carbohydrate intake and optimizing your health and weight loss goals. Here's how you can distinguish between the two:

1. Good Carbs (Low-Glycemic Carbs):

 - Non-Starchy Vegetables: These are rich in vitamins, minerals, and fiber while being low in carbs. Examples include leafy greens, broccoli, cauliflower, peppers, zucchini, and asparagus.

 - Low-Sugar Fruits: Choose fruits that are lower in sugar and higher in fiber, such as berries (strawberries, blueberries, raspberries), avocados, tomatoes, and lemons/limes. These fruits have a lower impact on blood sugar levels.

 - Whole Grains: Opt for whole grains that are minimally processed and high in fiber, such as oats, quinoa, barley, and brown rice. These provide sustained energy and essential nutrients.

2. Bad Carbs (High-Glycemic Carbs):

 - Refined Grains: These are grains that have been heavily processed and stripped of their fiber and nutrients. Examples include white bread, white rice, pasta, pastries, and most breakfast cereals.

 - Sugary Foods and Beverages: Avoid foods and drinks that are high in added sugars, such as candy, soda, fruit juices, sweetened yogurt, and desserts like cakes and cookies.

- Starchy Vegetables: Some vegetables are higher in carbohydrates and can spike blood sugar levels. Limit intake of starchy vegetables like potatoes, corn, peas, and winter squash on the Atkins diet.

3. Reading Labels:

- Check the nutrition labels of packaged foods to identify the carbohydrate content. Look for products with fewer grams of sugar and higher grams of fiber per serving.

- Pay attention to the ingredient list and avoid products with added sugars, refined grains, and ingredients you can't pronounce.

4. Understanding Glycemic Index (GI):

- Foods with a low glycemic index (GI) release glucose slowly into the bloodstream, helping to stabilize blood sugar levels. Aim to choose foods with a low GI whenever possible.

- Foods with a high GI cause rapid spikes in blood sugar levels, leading to energy crashes and cravings. These should be limited on the Atkins diet.

5. Portion Control:

- Even when consuming good carbs, it's important to practice portion control to manage your overall carbohydrate intake. Pay attention to serving sizes and avoid overeating, even with healthier carb options.

6. Balance and Moderation:

- While the Atkins diet emphasizes low-carb eating, it's important to remember that all carbohydrates can fit into a balanced diet when consumed in moderation.

- Focus on a variety of nutrient-dense foods, including lean proteins, healthy fats, and plenty of non-starchy vegetables, while being mindful of your carbohydrate intake.

Certainly! Here are some additional tips and insights to help you differentiate between good and bad carbs as an Atkins diet patient:

7. Understanding Net Carbs:

   - On the Atkins diet, focus on "net carbs," which is the total carbohydrate content minus the fiber content. Fiber is not fully absorbed by the body and has minimal impact on blood sugar levels. Tracking net carbs allows for a more accurate assessment of carbohydrate intake.

8. Lean Protein Emphasis:

   - Prioritize lean protein sources in your meals. Foods like poultry, fish, eggs, and tofu not only provide essential nutrients but also contribute to satiety, helping you feel full and satisfied.

9. Healthy Fats Inclusion:

   - Incorporate healthy fats into your diet, such as avocados, olive oil, nuts, and seeds. These fats contribute to a feeling of fullness and provide sustained energy without causing rapid spikes in blood sugar levels.

10. Beware of Hidden Sugars:

   - Be cautious of hidden sugars in processed foods, condiments, and sauces. Ingredients like high-fructose corn syrup, cane sugar, and other sweeteners can contribute to hidden carbs that may hinder your progress on the Atkins diet.

11. Meal Planning:

- Plan your meals in advance to ensure a balance of good carbs, proteins, and fats. This helps you avoid impulsive food choices and ensures that your meals align with the principles of the Atkins diet.

12. Consider Individual Tolerance:

- Understand your individual tolerance for carbs. Some people may be more sensitive to certain carbs than others. Pay attention to how your body responds to different foods and adjust your carb intake accordingly.

13. Educate Yourself on Food Labels:

- Learn how to interpret food labels accurately. Look for the total carbohydrate content, fiber content, and ingredient list. Avoid products with excessive added sugars, refined grains, and ingredients that are not in line with the Atkins diet.

14. Stay Hydrated with Water:

- Choose water as your primary beverage. Staying well-hydrated helps support overall health and can also contribute to a feeling of fullness, reducing the likelihood of overeating.

15. Explore Low-Carb Alternatives:

- Explore low-carb alternatives for your favorite foods. For example, use cauliflower rice instead of traditional rice, or lettuce wraps instead of tortillas. This allows you to enjoy familiar flavors while keeping your carb intake in check.

16. Regular Self-Monitoring:

- Regularly assess your progress and how your body responds to different foods. Keep a food diary or use a tracking app to monitor your daily food intake, allowing you to make informed adjustments to your diet.

17. Consult with a Dietitian:

- Consider consulting with a registered dietitian or nutritionist who specializes in low-carb diets. They can provide personalized guidance, help you understand your specific nutritional needs, and assist in creating a customized meal plan.

18. Lifestyle Integration:

- Integrate the principles of the Atkins diet into your lifestyle. Making it a long-term commitment rather than a short-term diet can help you sustain your success and make lasting changes to your eating habits.

<u>Reading food labels effectively</u>

Reading food labels effectively is crucial for Atkins diet patients to make informed choices about the foods they consume. Here's a guide to help you navigate food labels while following the Atkins diet:

1. Focus on Total Carbohydrates: Look at the total carbohydrate content listed on the food label. This includes all types of carbohydrates, including sugars, fiber, and starches. The Atkins diet emphasizes managing carbohydrate intake, so paying attention to this number is essential.

2. Calculate Net Carbs: Calculate the net carbs by subtracting the fiber content from the total carbohydrates. Net carbs represent the carbohydrates that have a significant impact on blood sugar levels. Since fiber is not fully absorbed by the

body, it has minimal impact on blood sugar and can be subtracted from the total carbs.

3. Consider Serving Size: Pay attention to the serving size listed on the food label. All of the nutrition information provided on the label is based on this serving size. Be mindful of portion sizes to accurately assess your carbohydrate intake.

4. Check the Ingredients List: Review the ingredients list to understand what's in the food product. Look for sources of added sugars, refined grains, and other high-carb ingredients that may not align with the Atkins diet. Ingredients are listed in descending order by weight, so those listed first are present in higher amounts.

5. Avoid Hidden Sugars: Be cautious of hidden sugars in processed foods. Ingredients like high-fructose corn syrup, cane sugar, and other sweeteners can contribute to hidden carbs that may hinder your progress on the Atkins diet.

6. Look for Whole Foods: Choose foods with minimal processing and recognizable ingredients. Whole foods like fruits, vegetables, lean proteins, and healthy fats are typically lower in carbs and higher in nutrients, making them ideal choices for the Atkins diet.

7. Check for Sugar Alcohols: Pay attention to sugar alcohols, which are often used as sweeteners in low-carb and sugar-free products. While sugar alcohols are lower in carbs than sugar, they can still have a significant impact on blood sugar levels for some individuals. Consider how your body responds to sugar alcohols and adjust your intake accordingly.

8. Be Wary of Claims: Be skeptical of health claims on food packaging, such as "low-fat" or "sugar-free." These claims can be misleading, and the product may still contain hidden carbs or other ingredients that are not conducive to the Atkins diet. Always refer to the nutrition label and ingredients list for accurate information.

9. Use a Tracking App: Consider using a smartphone app or online tool to track your daily food intake and monitor your carbohydrate intake. These tools can help you stay accountable and make informed choices about the foods you consume.

10. Educate Yourself: Take the time to educate yourself about common sources of carbohydrates and how to identify them on food labels. Familiarize yourself with terms like "sugar," "fiber," and "sugar alcohols" to better understand the nutritional content of the foods you eat.

11. Compare Similar Products: When choosing between similar products, compare their nutrition labels to identify the one with the lower carbohydrate content. Pay attention to differences in serving sizes and adjust accordingly to make a fair comparison.

12. Be Mindful of Portion Sizes: Keep in mind that the serving size listed on the food label may not always align with your portion size. Use measuring cups, spoons, or a food scale to accurately measure serving sizes, especially for foods that are easy to overeat, like nuts or granola.

13. Watch Out for Hidden Carbs: Be cautious of hidden sources of carbohydrates in seemingly low-carb foods. Ingredients like flour, cornstarch, maltodextrin, and

dextrose can add carbs to products that may not seem obvious. Pay attention to these ingredients, especially in packaged and processed foods.

14. Consider Glycemic Impact: In addition to total carbs, consider the glycemic impact of foods on your blood sugar levels. Some low-carb foods may still have a high glycemic index, leading to spikes in blood sugar levels. Choose foods with a lower glycemic index to help stabilize blood sugar levels.

15. Be Aware of "Low-Carb" Claims: Be cautious of products labeled as "low-carb" or "keto-friendly." While these products may have lower carbohydrate content than their regular counterparts, they may still contain ingredients that could stall your progress on the Atkins diet. Always check the nutrition label and ingredients list to verify their suitability for your dietary goals.

16. Check for Artificial Sweeteners: Watch out for artificial sweeteners like aspartame, sucralose, and saccharin, which are commonly used in low-carb and sugar-free products. While these sweeteners are low in carbs and calories, some people may experience negative effects or stalls in weight loss when consuming them. Pay attention to how your body responds and adjust your intake accordingly.

17. Read Allergen Information: If you have food allergies or sensitivities, carefully read the allergen information on food labels to ensure that the product is safe for you to consume. Common allergens like wheat, soy, and dairy may be present in unexpected places and can contribute to hidden carbs.

18. Be Prepared to Compare Labels: When shopping for groceries, be prepared to compare multiple options and read several food labels to find the best choices for

your dietary preferences. This may take extra time initially but will become easier with practice as you become more familiar with common ingredients and nutritional values.

19. Focus on Real, Whole Foods: Whenever possible, prioritize real, whole foods that don't require a nutrition label, such as fresh produce, lean proteins, and healthy fats. These foods are naturally low in carbs and provide essential nutrients, making them ideal choices for the Atkins diet.

<u>Managing sugar cravings and addiction</u>

Managing sugar cravings and overcoming sugar addiction can be challenging, but it's possible with the right strategies and mindset, especially as an Atkins diet patient. Here are some tips to help you manage sugar cravings and break free from sugar addiction while following the Atkins diet:

1. Understand the Science: Educate yourself about the effects of sugar on the body and why you may experience cravings. Sugar triggers the release of dopamine in the brain, creating feelings of pleasure and reward, which can contribute to cravings and addiction-like behavior.

2. Commit to the Atkins Diet: The Atkins diet focuses on reducing carbohydrate intake, including sugars, which can help minimize cravings over time. Commit to following the principles of the Atkins diet, including limiting sugar and processed carbs, to help manage cravings and break free from sugar addiction.

3. Gradually Reduce Sugar Intake: Instead of cutting out sugar cold turkey, gradually reduce your sugar intake over time. Start by eliminating the most

obvious sources of sugar, such as sugary beverages, desserts, and snacks, and gradually reduce your consumption of other high-sugar foods.

4. Choose Low-Carb Alternatives: Replace high-sugar foods with low-carb alternatives that satisfy your cravings without derailing your progress on the Atkins diet. For example, opt for sugar-free desserts sweetened with stevia or erythritol, or enjoy fresh fruit in moderation as a natural, low-sugar option.

5. Eat Balanced Meals: Ensure that your meals are balanced with a combination of protein, healthy fats, and fiber-rich carbohydrates from non-starchy vegetables. Eating balanced meals helps stabilize blood sugar levels and can reduce cravings for sugary foods.

6. Stay Hydrated: Drink plenty of water throughout the day to stay hydrated and reduce cravings. Sometimes thirst can be mistaken for hunger or sugar cravings, so staying hydrated can help curb the urge to reach for sugary snacks.

7. Include Protein and Healthy Fats: Include protein-rich foods and healthy fats in your meals and snacks to help keep you feeling satisfied and reduce cravings. Protein and fat help stabilize blood sugar levels and provide sustained energy, reducing the likelihood of sugar cravings.

8. Practice Mindful Eating: Pay attention to your hunger and fullness cues and practice mindful eating. Eat slowly, savor each bite, and tune in to how your body feels before, during, and after meals. Mindful eating can help you become more aware of your eating habits and reduce mindless snacking on sugary foods.

9. Manage Stress: Find healthy ways to manage stress, as stress can trigger cravings for sugary foods. Practice relaxation techniques such as deep breathing, meditation, yoga, or engaging in hobbies and activities that bring you joy and relaxation.

10. Get Adequate Sleep: Prioritize getting enough sleep each night, as sleep deprivation can disrupt hormones that regulate appetite and cravings. Aim for 7-9 hours of quality sleep per night to support overall health and reduce sugar cravings.

11. Identify Triggers: Identify your personal triggers for sugar cravings, such as stress, boredom, or emotional eating, and develop strategies to address them. Find alternative ways to cope with triggers, such as going for a walk, calling a friend, or practicing relaxation techniques.

12. Stay Consistent: Be consistent with your dietary choices and lifestyle habits, even when faced with occasional setbacks or cravings. Remember that progress takes time, and staying committed to the Atkins diet and healthy lifestyle choices will help you overcome sugar cravings and addiction in the long run.

13. Seek Support: Don't hesitate to seek support from friends, family, or a healthcare professional if you're struggling to manage sugar cravings or break free from sugar addiction. Having a support system can provide encouragement, accountability, and practical strategies for success.

14. Plan Balanced Snacks:

- Plan and prepare balanced snacks that align with the principles of the Atkins diet. Combining protein, healthy fats, and fiber-rich carbs in your snacks can help keep you satisfied and minimize the desire for sugary treats between meals.

15. Chew Sugar-Free Gum:

  - Chewing sugar-free gum can be a helpful way to occupy your mouth and reduce the desire for sweets. Look for gum sweetened with sugar alternatives like xylitol or stevia, keeping in mind that excessive consumption of sugar alcohols may impact some individuals differently.

16. Include Natural Sweeteners Sparingly:

  - While on the Atkins diet, you may choose to include natural sweeteners like stevia, erythritol, or monk fruit in moderation. Experiment with these alternatives in your recipes to add sweetness without the impact on blood sugar levels.

17. Create Sugar-Free Versions of Favorites:

  - Get creative in the kitchen and experiment with sugar-free versions of your favorite recipes. There are many low-carb and sugar-free alternatives for desserts and treats that can satisfy your sweet tooth while staying within the guidelines of the Atkins diet.

18. Practice Cognitive Behavioral Techniques:

  - Explore cognitive behavioral techniques to address the psychological aspects of sugar cravings. Identify and challenge negative thought patterns related to sugar, and replace them with positive affirmations and healthier coping mechanisms.

19. Stay Active:

- Engage in regular physical activity to help regulate blood sugar levels and reduce stress, both of which can contribute to sugar cravings. Choose activities you enjoy, whether it's walking, jogging, dancing, or participating in a fitness class.

20. Reward Non-Food Achievements:

- Find alternative ways to reward yourself for achievements or milestones that don't involve sugary treats. Treat yourself to a non-food reward such as a relaxing bath, a movie night, or a new book to reinforce positive behavior.

21. Practice Portion Control with Treats:

- If you decide to indulge in a sugary treat occasionally, practice portion control. Enjoy a small serving and savor the flavor, rather than consuming large quantities. This helps prevent feelings of guilt and minimizes the impact on your overall carb intake.

22. Use Visualization Techniques:

- Visualize your health and wellness goals to stay motivated and focused. Create mental images of how you want to feel and look, and use these positive visualizations to resist the temptation of sugary foods.

23. Keep Healthy Snacks Accessible:

- Keep healthy, low-carb snacks readily available to reduce the temptation of reaching for sugary options. Pre-cut vegetables, portioned nuts, and other convenient snacks can be a satisfying alternative when cravings strike.

24. Track Your Progress:

- Keep a journal or use a tracking app to record your progress, including your dietary choices, exercise routine, and any improvements in your overall well-being. Reflecting on your achievements can reinforce your commitment to the Atkins diet and help you stay on track.

25. Consider Professional Support:

- If sugar cravings persist or if you find it challenging to overcome sugar addiction, consider seeking support from a registered dietitian, nutritionist, or healthcare professional. They can provide personalized guidance, strategies, and encouragement to help you navigate and overcome challenges.

Chapter 8 : The Science Behind the Atkins Diet

How the body metabolizes carbohydrates

As an Atkins diet patient, understanding how the body metabolizes carbohydrates is crucial for optimizing your dietary choices and achieving your health and weight loss goals. Here's a breakdown of how the body metabolizes carbohydrates on the Atkins diet:

1. Digestion Begins in the Mouth: The process of carbohydrate metabolism begins as soon as you start chewing food. Carbohydrates are broken down into simpler sugars like glucose, maltose, and sucrose through the action of enzymes in saliva, particularly amylase.

2. Stomach Digestion: Once in the stomach, carbohydrates continue to be broken down by stomach acid and digestive enzymes. However, the primary digestion of carbohydrates occurs in the small intestine.

3. Small Intestine Absorption: In the small intestine, carbohydrates are further broken down into their simplest form, such as glucose, fructose, and galactose. These simple sugars are then absorbed into the bloodstream through the lining of the small intestine.

4. Blood Sugar Regulation: When carbohydrates are absorbed into the bloodstream, they cause blood sugar levels to rise. In response, the pancreas releases insulin, a hormone that helps move glucose from the bloodstream into cells for energy or storage.

5. Cellular Energy Production: Inside the cells, glucose is either used immediately for energy or stored as glycogen in the liver and muscles for later use. When glycogen stores are full, excess glucose is converted into fat for long-term energy storage.

6. Insulin Response: On the Atkins diet, which is low in carbohydrates, blood sugar levels remain relatively stable due to reduced carbohydrate intake. This results in lower insulin levels, as less insulin is needed to regulate blood sugar.

7. Shift to Fat Burning: With reduced carbohydrate intake and lower insulin levels, the body shifts to burning fat for fuel, a process known as ketosis. In ketosis, the liver produces ketones from fat stores, which can be used as an alternative fuel source by the brain and other tissues.

8. Glycogen Depletion: During the initial phases of the Atkins diet, glycogen stores are depleted as carbohydrate intake is restricted. This leads to a rapid decrease in water weight due to the loss of glycogen-associated water.

9. Carbohydrate Reintroduction: As the Atkins diet progresses through its phases, carbohydrates are gradually reintroduced in controlled amounts. This allows for the replenishment of glycogen stores without causing significant fluctuations in blood sugar levels or disrupting ketosis.

10. Individual Variations: It's important to note that the body's response to carbohydrate metabolism can vary among individuals. Factors such as metabolism, insulin sensitivity, activity level, and overall health can influence how carbohydrates are metabolized and utilized for energy.

Certainly! Here are some additional details about how the body metabolizes carbohydrates for an Atkins diet patient:

11. Gluconeogenesis: In the absence of dietary carbohydrates, the body can produce glucose through a process called gluconeogenesis. During gluconeogenesis, certain amino acids, lactate, and glycerol are converted into glucose in the liver. This helps maintain blood sugar levels and provides a source of energy for tissues that rely on glucose, such as red blood cells and certain parts of the brain.

12. Role of Ketones: As carbohydrate intake is reduced on the Atkins diet, the body transitions into a state of ketosis, where ketone bodies become the primary source of fuel for many tissues, including the brain. Ketones are produced by the liver from fatty acids when glycogen stores are depleted and blood glucose levels are low. This metabolic state allows the body to efficiently burn fat for energy and can lead to weight loss.

13. Steady Energy Levels: By limiting carbohydrate intake and stabilizing blood sugar levels, the Atkins diet helps prevent the energy crashes and cravings associated with high-carbohydrate meals. Instead, individuals on the Atkins diet may experience steady energy levels throughout the day, without the fluctuations in energy commonly observed with high-carb diets.

14. Improved Insulin Sensitivity: Research suggests that low-carbohydrate diets like Atkins may improve insulin sensitivity and reduce insulin resistance in individuals with obesity and type 2 diabetes. By minimizing fluctuations in blood

sugar and insulin levels, the Atkins diet can help improve metabolic health and support weight loss.

15. Satiety and Appetite Regulation: The high protein and fat content of the Atkins diet can help increase feelings of fullness and satiety, leading to reduced calorie intake and improved appetite regulation. Protein and fat take longer to digest compared to carbohydrates, helping to prolong feelings of fullness and reduce the urge to snack between meals.

16. Maintenance of Muscle Mass: Adequate protein intake on the Atkins diet helps support muscle maintenance and repair, even during periods of carbohydrate restriction. This is important for preserving lean body mass and metabolic rate, which can help prevent weight regain and support long-term weight management.

17. Customization for Individual Needs: One of the benefits of the Atkins diet is its flexibility and adaptability to individual preferences and needs. The diet can be customized based on factors such as activity level, metabolic health, and weight loss goals. This allows for personalized carbohydrate intake levels that optimize metabolic health and weight loss success.

18. Long-Term Sustainability: Some individuals find that the Atkins diet is easier to sustain long-term compared to traditional low-fat, high-carb diets. The emphasis on whole, nutrient-dense foods, along with the flexibility to gradually reintroduce carbohydrates as tolerated, can make the Atkins diet a sustainable lifestyle choice for many people.

Impact of insulin on fat storage and energy levels

Insulin plays a crucial role in regulating fat storage and energy levels in the body. Here's an overview of how insulin impacts these processes:

1. Glucose Uptake and Storage:

   - When you consume carbohydrates, they are broken down into glucose, leading to an increase in blood sugar levels. In response to elevated blood glucose, the pancreas releases insulin into the bloodstream.

2. Insulin and Glucose Transport:

   - Insulin acts as a key that unlocks the cells, allowing glucose to enter. This is especially important for cells that require glucose for energy, such as muscle cells. Insulin facilitates the transport of glucose from the bloodstream into cells.

3. Glycogen Synthesis:

   - In addition to promoting glucose uptake by cells, insulin stimulates the conversion of excess glucose into glycogen in the liver and muscles. Glycogen serves as a stored form of glucose, readily available for energy when needed.

4. Fat Storage (Lipogenesis):

   - When insulin levels are elevated, the body shifts its focus toward storing excess energy. Insulin promotes lipogenesis, a process where excess glucose is converted into fatty acids and stored as triglycerides in fat cells (adipocytes).

5. Inhibition of Lipolysis:

   - Insulin inhibits lipolysis, which is the breakdown of stored fat into fatty acids for energy. When insulin levels are high, the body prioritizes using glucose for energy and suppresses the release of fatty acids from fat stores.

6. Effects on Appetite and Satiety:

- Insulin also influences feelings of hunger and fullness. Elevated insulin levels after a meal can contribute to feelings of satiety, signaling to the body that it has received sufficient energy.

7. Role in Energy Storage:

- Insulin is a key player in the body's energy storage mechanisms. It facilitates the storage of excess nutrients during periods of plenty, ensuring a readily available energy source for times of scarcity or increased energy demand.

8. Insulin Sensitivity:

- Insulin sensitivity refers to how efficiently cells respond to insulin's signals. High insulin sensitivity is associated with effective glucose uptake and lower risk of insulin resistance. Insulin resistance, on the other hand, occurs when cells become less responsive to insulin, leading to elevated blood sugar levels.

9. Impact on Energy Levels:

- While insulin helps store excess energy, it can also influence energy levels. After consuming a high-carbohydrate meal, insulin facilitates the uptake of glucose into cells, providing a quick source of energy. However, this energy surge is often followed by a dip in blood sugar levels, potentially leading to feelings of fatigue or hunger.

10. Metabolic Health:

- Chronic elevation of insulin levels, often associated with a diet high in refined carbohydrates and added sugars, can contribute to metabolic imbalances. Over time, insulin resistance may develop, leading to difficulties in effectively managing blood sugar levels and increased risk of type 2 diabetes.

Certainly! Here are some additional insights into the impact of insulin on fat storage and energy levels:

11. Feedback Loop with Blood Sugar:

   - Insulin secretion is tightly regulated by blood sugar levels. When blood sugar rises after a meal, insulin is released to help transport glucose into cells for energy or storage. This process helps maintain blood sugar within a narrow range, preventing it from reaching dangerously high levels (hyperglycemia).

12. Fat Storage and Weight Gain:

   - Elevated insulin levels, particularly in response to a high-carbohydrate diet, can promote fat storage and weight gain over time. When insulin levels are chronically elevated, as is common in individuals with insulin resistance or type 2 diabetes, the body may store more fat, especially around the abdomen (visceral fat).

13. Role in Lipogenesis:

   - Insulin promotes lipogenesis, the conversion of excess glucose into fatty acids, which are then stored as triglycerides in fat cells. This process occurs primarily in the liver and adipose tissue. Elevated insulin levels can lead to increased fat accumulation, contributing to weight gain and obesity.

14. Insulin Resistance and Metabolic Syndrome:

   - Insulin resistance occurs when cells become less responsive to the effects of insulin, leading to elevated blood sugar levels and compensatory increases in insulin secretion. Insulin resistance is a hallmark of metabolic syndrome, a cluster of conditions that increase the risk of heart disease, type 2 diabetes, and other health problems.

15. Impact on Energy Expenditure:

- While insulin promotes the storage of excess energy as fat, it can also influence energy expenditure. Elevated insulin levels may suppress the breakdown of stored fat (lipolysis) for energy, leading to reduced fat utilization and potentially contributing to feelings of fatigue or lethargy.

16. Effects on Hormone Regulation:

- Insulin interacts with other hormones involved in metabolism, such as leptin (which regulates appetite and energy expenditure) and ghrelin (which stimulates hunger). Dysregulation of these hormonal signals, often associated with insulin resistance, can disrupt appetite control and contribute to weight gain.

17. Exercise and Insulin Sensitivity:

- Regular physical activity, particularly aerobic exercise and resistance training, can improve insulin sensitivity and help mitigate the negative effects of insulin resistance. Exercise enhances glucose uptake by muscle cells, reducing the reliance on insulin for glucose disposal and improving overall metabolic health.

18. Dietary Strategies for Managing Insulin Levels:

- Certain dietary strategies can help manage insulin levels and promote metabolic health. These include reducing intake of refined carbohydrates and added sugars, increasing consumption of fiber-rich foods, choosing nutrient-dense whole foods, and incorporating sources of healthy fats and lean proteins into meals.

19. Individual Variability:

- It's important to recognize that individual responses to insulin can vary based on factors such as genetics, age, body composition, and overall health status. Some individuals may be more sensitive to the effects of insulin, while others may experience insulin resistance and its associated metabolic consequences.

20. Consultation with Healthcare Professionals:

- For individuals with concerns about insulin resistance, metabolic health, or weight management, consulting with healthcare professionals, such as a registered dietitian, endocrinologist, or primary care physician, can provide personalized guidance and support for optimizing insulin sensitivity and overall health.

Research supporting the Atkins approach

The Atkins diet, developed by Dr. Robert Atkins in the 1970s, has been the subject of numerous research studies investigating its efficacy for weight loss, metabolic health, and various health outcomes. While some earlier studies raised concerns about the diet's high-fat content and potential cardiovascular risks, more recent research has provided evidence supporting the Atkins approach. Here's an overview of research supporting the Atkins diet:

1. Weight Loss and Fat Loss:

- Several studies have demonstrated that the Atkins diet is effective for promoting weight loss and reducing body fat. A meta-analysis published in the British Journal of Nutrition in 2006 found that low-carbohydrate diets, including the Atkins diet, were associated with significantly greater weight loss compared to low-fat diets over a period of six months to two years.

2. Metabolic Benefits:

   - Research has shown that the Atkins diet can lead to improvements in various metabolic markers, including blood sugar levels, insulin sensitivity, and lipid profiles. A study published in the Annals of Internal Medicine in 2004 found that overweight and obese individuals following a low-carbohydrate diet like Atkins experienced greater improvements in insulin sensitivity and triglyceride levels compared to those following a low-fat diet.

3. Appetite Regulation:

   - Some studies have suggested that the Atkins diet may have favorable effects on appetite regulation, leading to reduced calorie intake and increased satiety. Research published in JAMA Internal Medicine in 2014 found that individuals following a low-carbohydrate diet reported greater reductions in hunger and cravings compared to those on a low-fat diet, which may contribute to long-term adherence and weight loss success.

4. Cardiovascular Risk Factors:

   - While early concerns were raised about the potential cardiovascular risks of the Atkins diet due to its high-fat content, more recent research has suggested that the diet may have neutral or even beneficial effects on cardiovascular risk factors. A meta-analysis published in the Journal of the American College of Cardiology in 2019 found that low-carbohydrate diets were associated with improvements in several cardiovascular risk factors, including blood pressure, triglycerides, and HDL cholesterol levels.

5. Sustainability and Adherence:

- Research has also examined the sustainability and long-term adherence of the Atkins diet compared to other dietary approaches. A study published in the New England Journal of Medicine in 2003 found that overweight individuals following a low-carbohydrate diet like Atkins were more likely to adhere to the diet and achieve greater weight loss compared to those following a low-fat diet over a period of one year.

6. Potential Benefits for Specific Populations:

- Some research has explored the potential benefits of the Atkins diet for specific populations, such as individuals with type 2 diabetes or metabolic syndrome. A study published in Diabetes Care in 2008 found that overweight individuals with type 2 diabetes following a low-carbohydrate diet experienced greater improvements in glycemic control and medication reduction compared to those on a low-fat diet.

7. Individualized Approach:

- One of the strengths of the Atkins approach is its flexibility and adaptability to individual preferences and needs. Research has suggested that personalized dietary approaches, including low-carbohydrate diets like Atkins, may be more effective for long-term weight management and metabolic health compared to one-size-fits-all dietary recommendations.

Certainly! Here are some additional insights into the research supporting the Atkins approach:

8. Effectiveness for Insulin Resistance and Type 2 Diabetes:

- Research has shown that the Atkins diet may be particularly beneficial for individuals with insulin resistance and type 2 diabetes. A study published in

Diabetes, Obesity & Metabolism in 2011 found that a low-carbohydrate, ketogenic diet like Atkins improved glycemic control, reduced medication use, and led to greater weight loss compared to a low-glycemic, reduced-calorie diet in overweight individuals with type 2 diabetes.

9. Effects on Blood Sugar Levels:

   - The Atkins diet has been shown to have favorable effects on blood sugar levels, particularly in individuals with insulin resistance or prediabetes. A study published in Nutrition & Metabolism in 2008 found that overweight individuals following a low-carbohydrate diet experienced greater reductions in fasting blood glucose and hemoglobin A1c levels compared to those on a low-fat diet.

10. Impact on Cardiovascular Risk Factors:

   - While earlier concerns were raised about the potential impact of the Atkins diet on cardiovascular risk factors, recent research suggests that the diet may have neutral or even beneficial effects on certain cardiovascular risk markers. A study published in the Journal of the American College of Cardiology in 2010 found that a low-carbohydrate diet improved several cardiovascular risk factors, including high-sensitivity C-reactive protein (hs-CRP) levels and triglyceride-HDL cholesterol ratio, compared to a low-fat diet in overweight and obese women.

11. Long-Term Sustainability:

   - Some research has examined the long-term sustainability and adherence of the Atkins diet compared to other dietary approaches. A study published in Obesity Research in 2005 found that overweight individuals following a low-carbohydrate diet like Atkins maintained greater weight loss and improvements in metabolic markers compared to those following a low-fat diet over a period of two years.

12. Potential Mechanisms of Action:

- Research has explored the potential mechanisms underlying the effectiveness of the Atkins diet, including its effects on appetite regulation, metabolic flexibility, and hormonal signaling. Some studies suggest that the low-carbohydrate, high-protein, and high-fat nature of the Atkins diet may promote satiety, increase thermogenesis, and improve insulin sensitivity, contributing to weight loss and metabolic improvements.

13. Comparison to Other Dietary Approaches:

- Several studies have compared the Atkins diet to other popular dietary approaches, such as the Mediterranean diet, low-fat diet, and low-glycemic diet. While results vary depending on the study population and outcomes measured, some research suggests that the Atkins diet may be equally or more effective for weight loss and improving metabolic health compared to other dietary approaches in certain populations.

14. Considerations for Individualization:

- It's important to recognize that the effectiveness of the Atkins diet may vary depending on individual factors such as genetics, metabolic health, lifestyle factors, and personal preferences. Some individuals may thrive on a low-carbohydrate diet like Atkins, while others may prefer or respond better to different dietary approaches. Personalization and individualization are key considerations when implementing the Atkins approach or any dietary plan.

Chapter 9: Frequently Asked Questions

Addressing common concerns and misconceptions

Certainly! Here are answers to some frequently asked questions about the Atkins diet:

1. What is the Atkins Diet?

   - The Atkins diet is a low-carbohydrate diet designed for weight loss and improved overall health. It emphasizes reducing carb intake to achieve a state of ketosis, where the body burns fat for fuel.

2. How Does the Atkins Diet Work?

   - The Atkins diet works by restricting carbohydrate intake, leading the body to burn stored fat for energy. It is divided into phases, starting with induction (very low carb) and gradually reintroducing carbs as weight loss goals are met.

3. What Can I Eat on the Atkins Diet?

   - Allowed foods include meat, fish, eggs, low-carb vegetables, full-fat dairy, and healthy fats. Foods to limit or avoid include grains, sugary foods, fruits, and high-carb processed foods.

4. Is the Atkins Diet Suitable for Everyone?

   - The Atkins diet may not be suitable for everyone, especially those with certain medical conditions. Individuals with kidney problems, for example, should consult a healthcare professional before starting the diet.

5. Can I Exercise on the Atkins Diet?

- Yes, exercise is encouraged on the Atkins diet. Regular physical activity can enhance weight loss, improve metabolic health, and support overall well-being.

6. How Long Does Each Phase of the Atkins Diet Last?

- The duration of each phase varies. The Induction phase typically lasts two weeks or longer, while subsequent phases depend on individual weight loss goals and how the body responds to carb reintroduction.

7. Can I Follow the Atkins Diet as a Vegetarian or Vegan?

- While challenging, it is possible to adapt the Atkins diet for vegetarians or vegans. Protein sources such as tofu, tempeh, and plant-based protein sources can be included.

8. Will I Experience Ketosis on the Atkins Diet?

- Yes, ketosis is a key aspect of the Atkins diet, particularly during the Induction phase. This is when the body shifts to burning fat for energy and produces ketones.

9. Are There Risks Associated with the Atkins Diet?

- Some individuals may experience side effects like the "keto flu" during the initial stages. Long-term risks may include nutrient deficiencies if the diet is not well-balanced. Consulting a healthcare professional is advisable.

10. Can I Drink Alcohol on the Atkins Diet?

- Some low-carb alcoholic beverages may be allowed, but alcohol intake should be moderated. Alcohol can slow down weight loss and affect ketosis.

11. What Are the Common Pitfalls on the Atkins Diet?

- Common pitfalls include inadequate hydration, not eating enough vegetables, and relying too heavily on processed low-carb products. It's crucial to prioritize nutrient-dense, whole foods.

12. Is the Atkins Diet Sustainable for the Long Term?

- The sustainability of the Atkins diet varies among individuals. Some find it sustainable as a long-term lifestyle, while others may prefer more flexibility in their dietary choices.

13. Can I Do the Atkins Diet While Pregnant or Breastfeeding?

- Pregnancy and breastfeeding require additional nutrients. Consult a healthcare professional before making significant dietary changes during these periods.

14. Can I Follow the Atkins Diet if I Have Diabetes?

- The Atkins diet may be suitable for some individuals with diabetes, but close monitoring of blood sugar levels and consultation with a healthcare professional is essential.

15. How Quickly Can I Expect to See Results on the Atkins Diet?

- Weight loss varies, but some individuals may experience rapid weight loss, especially during the initial phases. Results depend on factors like adherence, metabolism, and individual response.

Addressing common concerns and misconceptions of the Atkins diet is important for providing accurate information and helping individuals make informed decisions about their dietary choices. Here are some common concerns and misconceptions about the Atkins diet, along with explanations to address them:

1. Misconception: The Atkins diet is unhealthy because it encourages high-fat consumption.

   - Addressing Concern: While the Atkins diet does emphasize higher fat intake compared to traditional low-fat diets, it focuses on healthy fats such as those found in avocados, nuts, seeds, and olive oil. Research suggests that healthy fats can have beneficial effects on heart health and overall well-being when consumed as part of a balanced diet.

2. Misconception: The Atkins diet is all about eating unlimited amounts of meat and cheese.

   - Addressing Concern: While protein-rich foods like meat and cheese are included in the Atkins diet, it also emphasizes non-starchy vegetables, healthy fats, and nutrient-dense foods. The diet encourages a balanced approach to nutrition, and portion control is important for achieving weight loss and overall health goals.

3. Misconception: The Atkins diet eliminates all carbohydrates, including fruits and vegetables.

   - Addressing Concern: The Atkins diet does restrict carbohydrate intake, particularly during the initial phases, but it emphasizes nutrient-dense carbohydrates from non-starchy vegetables. Low-carb fruits such as berries can also be included in moderation. The diet encourages choosing whole, unprocessed foods to meet nutrient needs.

4. Misconception: The Atkins diet is a fad diet that promotes quick fixes and unsustainable weight loss.

- Addressing Concern: While the Atkins diet has been criticized as a fad diet in the past, research suggests that it can be effective for sustainable weight loss and improving metabolic health when followed properly. The diet offers a structured approach to carbohydrate restriction and emphasizes long-term lifestyle changes rather than short-term fixes.

5. Misconception: The Atkins diet can lead to nutrient deficiencies due to its restrictive nature.

- Addressing Concern: Like any diet, it's important to ensure adequate nutrient intake on the Atkins diet. While carbohydrate intake is restricted, the diet encourages consumption of nutrient-dense foods such as vegetables, nuts, seeds, and healthy fats. Supplementation or careful meal planning may be necessary to ensure adequate intake of certain nutrients, especially during the initial phases.

6. Misconception: The Atkins diet causes constipation due to low fiber intake.

- Addressing Concern: While low-carb diets may initially lead to lower fiber intake, the Atkins diet encourages consumption of fiber-rich vegetables, nuts, seeds, and low-carb fruits to support digestive health. Adequate hydration and regular physical activity can also help prevent constipation while following the diet.

7. Misconception: The Atkins diet increases the risk of heart disease due to its high-fat content.

- Addressing Concern: Research on the long-term effects of the Atkins diet on heart health has yielded mixed results. While some studies suggest that the diet may have neutral or beneficial effects on cardiovascular risk factors, others have raised concerns about its potential impact on cholesterol levels. It's important to monitor cholesterol levels and consult with a healthcare professional if necessary while following the Atkins diet.

8. Misconception: The Atkins diet is only effective for short-term weight loss and is not sustainable in the long run.

   - Addressing Concern: Research suggests that the Atkins diet can be effective for both short-term weight loss and long-term weight maintenance when followed properly. The diet offers flexibility in its approach to carbohydrate restriction and encourages gradual reintroduction of carbs based on individual tolerance and weight loss goals. Long-term adherence to the diet may require ongoing support and guidance from healthcare professionals or registered dietitians.

9. Misconception: The Atkins diet is too restrictive, making it difficult to follow.

   - Addressing Concern: While the initial phases of the Atkins diet involve stricter carbohydrate restriction, the diet becomes more flexible over time. The approach encourages individuals to find a sustainable level of carbohydrate intake that aligns with their health goals. This adaptability can make the diet more feasible for long-term adherence.

10. Misconception: The Atkins diet may lead to muscle loss due to the emphasis on protein.

   - Addressing Concern: Adequate protein intake is a key aspect of the Atkins diet, and it's important for supporting muscle maintenance and overall health. The diet aims to preserve lean body mass, especially during weight loss, by providing sufficient protein. Regular resistance training exercises can further help maintain muscle mass.

11. Misconception: The Atkins diet is not suitable for athletes or those with high activity levels.

- Addressing Concern: The Atkins diet can be adapted for individuals with high activity levels, including athletes. Adjustments in carbohydrate intake can be made based on energy needs and training intensity. Carbohydrate cycling, where higher carb days align with intense workouts, is one approach to accommodate athletic performance while following the Atkins diet.

12. Misconception: The Atkins diet can lead to an increase in cholesterol levels.

- Addressing Concern: Research on the impact of the Atkins diet on cholesterol levels has shown mixed results. While some studies suggest an increase in LDL cholesterol (considered "bad" cholesterol) for some individuals, others indicate improvements in the overall cholesterol profile. It's important to monitor cholesterol levels regularly and consult with a healthcare professional for personalized guidance.

13. Misconception: The Atkins diet neglects the importance of fruits and whole grains.

- Addressing Concern: While the Atkins diet limits certain fruits and whole grains during the initial phases, it encourages the reintroduction of these foods in later phases. The focus is on choosing nutrient-dense, low-carb options. Incorporating a variety of colorful vegetables and low-carb fruits ensures a diverse range of vitamins, minerals, and antioxidants.

14. Misconception: The Atkins diet lacks fiber, leading to digestive issues.

- Addressing Concern: The Atkins diet emphasizes non-starchy vegetables, nuts, seeds, and low-carb fruits, which contribute to fiber intake. Adequate hydration and the inclusion of fiber supplements or low-carb alternatives can further support digestive health. Balancing fiber sources is crucial for preventing constipation.

15. Misconception: The Atkins diet may cause energy crashes and fatigue.

- Addressing Concern: While individuals may experience an adjustment period known as the "keto flu" during the initial phases, energy levels often stabilize as the body adapts to using fat for fuel. Ensuring sufficient intake of healthy fats, staying hydrated, and gradually adjusting to the diet can help minimize energy fluctuations.

16. Misconception: The Atkins diet is not suitable for older adults.

- Addressing Concern: The Atkins diet can be adapted for individuals of various ages, including older adults. However, personalized considerations such as medical history, nutritional needs, and individual health conditions should be taken into account. Consulting with a healthcare professional is advisable for personalized guidance.

17. Misconception: The Atkins diet promotes an unhealthy focus on weight loss rather than overall well-being.

- Addressing Concern: While weight loss is a common goal of the Atkins diet, it also emphasizes overall well-being and metabolic health. The diet encourages the consumption of nutrient-dense foods, regular physical activity, and long-term lifestyle changes for sustainable health benefits beyond weight loss.

18. Misconception: The Atkins diet may lead to social isolation due to dietary restrictions.

- Addressing Concern: The Atkins diet can be adapted to social situations by making informed choices and communicating dietary preferences. Planning ahead, choosing low-carb options at social events, and explaining dietary choices to others can help individuals follow the diet while remaining socially engaged.

Troubleshooting common issues

Troubleshooting common issues as an Atkins diet patient involves addressing challenges that may arise during the course of following the diet. Here are some common issues and strategies to troubleshoot them:

1. Issue: Feeling Fatigued or Lethargic

   - Troubleshooting: Ensure you are consuming an adequate amount of healthy fats for energy. Consider adjusting your macronutrient ratios to find the right balance for your energy needs. Stay well-hydrated and consider incorporating electrolyte-rich foods or supplements, especially during the initial phases.

2. Issue: Difficulty with Digestion or Constipation

   - Troubleshooting: Increase your intake of non-starchy vegetables, nuts, seeds, and low-carb fruits to boost fiber intake. Stay hydrated by drinking plenty of water throughout the day. Consider adding sources of healthy fats like avocados or olive oil to support digestive health.

3. Issue: Plateau in Weight Loss

   - Troubleshooting: Reevaluate your portion sizes and daily caloric intake. Track your food intake to identify any hidden carbs or excessive calorie consumption. Incorporate variety in your meals and consider adjusting your carbohydrate intake within the recommended range. Adding more physical activity or changing the type of exercise may also help overcome a weight loss plateau.

4. Issue: Social Challenges or Dining Out

   - Troubleshooting: Plan ahead when attending social events or dining out. Research restaurant menus in advance and choose low-carb options. Communicate your dietary preferences to friends and family to avoid potential misunderstandings. Focus on enjoying social interactions rather than solely on the food.

5. Issue: Sweet Cravings or Emotional Eating

   - Troubleshooting: Choose low-carb alternatives for sweet cravings, such as sugar-free desserts or berries. Identify and address emotional triggers for eating. Practice mindful eating, and if cravings persist, consider consulting with a registered dietitian for personalized strategies.

6. Issue: Difficulty Adapting to Ketosis

   - Troubleshooting: Gradually reduce carbohydrate intake during the initial phases to allow your body to adapt. Stay hydrated and consume adequate electrolytes. Incorporate healthy fats to support ketone production. Be patient, as it may take some time for your body to transition into ketosis.

7. Issue: Lack of Variety in Meals

   - Troubleshooting: Explore new recipes and experiment with different low-carb ingredients to add variety to your meals. Include a diverse range of vegetables, proteins, and fats. Plan your meals in advance to avoid falling into a routine, and consider incorporating seasonings and spices for flavor.

8. Issue: Feeling Overwhelmed or Stressed

   - Troubleshooting: Break down your goals into manageable steps. Seek support from friends, family, or online communities following similar dietary patterns. Consider consulting with a healthcare professional or a registered dietitian for guidance and personalized strategies. Practice stress-reducing techniques such as mindfulness or meditation.

9. Issue: Concerns About Nutrient Deficiencies

   - Troubleshooting: Ensure you are consuming a variety of nutrient-dense foods. Consider incorporating a multivitamin or specific supplements as recommended by a healthcare professional. Regularly monitor your nutrient intake and adjust your diet if needed.

10. Issue: Lack of Motivation or Boredom

   - Troubleshooting: Set realistic and achievable goals to maintain motivation. Celebrate small successes along the way. Keep your meals interesting by trying new recipes and experimenting with different food combinations. Consider finding a diet buddy or joining a community for mutual support.

11. Issue: Irregular Bowel Movements

   - Troubleshooting: Ensure you are consuming enough fiber from low-carb vegetables, nuts, and seeds. Adequate hydration is crucial for maintaining regular bowel movements. If constipation persists, consider adding magnesium-rich foods or supplements, as magnesium can have a laxative effect.

12. Issue: Increased Hunger or Appetite

- Troubleshooting: Reevaluate your portion sizes and the distribution of macronutrients in your meals. Ensure you are consuming enough healthy fats and protein to promote satiety. If hunger persists, consider adjusting your daily caloric intake or incorporating more fiber-rich foods.

13. Issue: Inconsistent Energy Levels

- Troubleshooting:** Monitor your carbohydrate intake and adjust it to align with your energy needs. Spread your meals throughout the day to maintain stable blood sugar levels. Consider adding nutrient-dense snacks, such as cheese or raw vegetables, to sustain energy between meals.

14. Issue: Difficulty Sticking to the Plan

- Troubleshooting: Revisit your goals and remind yourself of the reasons you chose the Atkins diet. Focus on the positive changes you've experienced and the benefits of the diet for your health. Seek support from friends, family, or online communities. Consider consulting with a healthcare professional or a registered dietitian for personalized guidance.

15. Issue: Challenges with Exercise Performance

- Troubleshooting: Ensure you are consuming enough calories, especially from healthy fats, to support your energy needs during exercise. Consider adjusting your carbohydrate intake around workouts, consuming a small amount of easily digestible carbs before exercise if needed. Experiment with the timing and type of exercise to find what works best for you.

16. Issue: Insomnia or Disrupted Sleep

- Troubleshooting:** Monitor your caffeine intake, especially in the evening, as it can interfere with sleep. Ensure you are getting enough magnesium, which plays a role in sleep regulation. Establish a consistent sleep routine and create a calming environment before bedtime.

17. Issue: Concerns About Cholesterol Levels

- Troubleshooting: If you have concerns about cholesterol levels, consult with a healthcare professional. Consider incorporating heart-healthy fats, such as those found in avocados and fatty fish. Regularly monitor your cholesterol levels, and if needed, explore dietary adjustments under the guidance of a healthcare professional.

18. Issue: Traveling While on the Atkins Diet

- Troubleshooting: Plan ahead by researching food options at your destination and packing low-carb snacks. Choose protein-rich options at restaurants and focus on whole, unprocessed foods. Stay hydrated, especially during air travel, to prevent dehydration.

19. Issue: Feeling Socially Isolated

- Troubleshooting: Communicate your dietary preferences to friends and family to foster understanding. Bring a low-carb dish to social events. Seek out support groups or online communities of individuals following similar dietary patterns for encouragement and shared experiences.

20. Issue: Concerns About Sustainability

- Troubleshooting:** Focus on creating a flexible and sustainable version of the Atkins diet that works for your lifestyle. Experiment with different recipes and meal plans to keep your meals interesting. Regularly reassess your dietary choices and make adjustments as needed to meet your evolving goals.

<u>Tips for long-term success and maintenance</u>

Achieving long-term success and maintenance on the Atkins diet involves adopting sustainable lifestyle habits and making informed choices that support your health and well-being. Here are some tips for long-term success and maintenance as an Atkins diet patient:

1. Focus on Whole Foods: Emphasize whole, unprocessed foods in your diet, including lean proteins, non-starchy vegetables, healthy fats, and low-carb fruits. Choose nutrient-dense options to support overall health and well-being.

2. Stay Hydrated: Drink plenty of water throughout the day to stay hydrated. Adequate hydration supports digestion, metabolism, and overall health. Aim for at least 8-10 glasses of water per day, or more if you are physically active.

3. Monitor Portion Sizes: Pay attention to portion sizes to prevent overeating and support weight management. Use measuring cups, spoons, or food scales to accurately measure serving sizes, especially during the initial phases of the Atkins diet.

4. Practice Mindful Eating: Be mindful of your eating habits and pay attention to hunger and satiety cues. Eat slowly, savoring each bite, and stop when you feel satisfied. Avoid distractions such as television or electronic devices while eating.

5. Incorporate Regular Physical Activity: Include regular physical activity in your routine to support overall health and weight management. Aim for a combination of aerobic exercise, strength training, and flexibility exercises. Find activities you enjoy to make exercise a sustainable part of your lifestyle.

6. Plan and Prepare Meals: Plan your meals and snacks in advance to avoid impulsive food choices. Batch cook and meal prep to have healthy options readily available throughout the week. Stock your kitchen with low-carb staples to support your dietary goals.

7. Seek Support and Accountability: Connect with a support system of friends, family, or online communities following similar dietary patterns. Share your goals, challenges, and successes with others for encouragement and accountability. Consider joining a support group or working with a registered dietitian for personalized guidance.

8. Be Flexible and Adaptable: Be flexible in your approach to the Atkins diet and willing to adjust as needed based on your individual preferences and lifestyle. Experiment with different recipes, meal plans, and food combinations to keep your meals interesting and enjoyable.

9. Manage Stress: Incorporate stress-reducing techniques such as mindfulness, meditation, deep breathing exercises, or yoga into your daily routine. Chronic stress can affect appetite, food choices, and overall health, so prioritize activities that promote relaxation and well-being.

10. Regularly Monitor Progress: Track your progress by monitoring key metrics such as weight, body measurements, energy levels, and overall well-being. Regularly reassess your dietary choices and lifestyle habits to ensure they align with your long-term goals.

11. Celebrate Successes: Celebrate your achievements and milestones along the way. Acknowledge your progress, no matter how small, and reward yourself with non-food rewards that support your overall well-being.

12. Stay Informed: Stay informed about the latest research and developments related to the Atkins diet and low-carb nutrition. Keep learning and seeking out reliable sources of information to support your long-term success and maintenance. Certainly! Here are additional tips to support long-term success and maintenance as an Atkins diet patient:

13. Practice Self-Compassion: Be kind to yourself and recognize that achieving long-term success on the Atkins diet is a journey. Embrace the ups and downs, and avoid being too hard on yourself if you experience setbacks. Focus on progress rather than perfection, and celebrate your efforts along the way.

14. Listen to Your Body: Pay attention to how different foods make you feel and how your body responds to the Atkins diet. Tune in to hunger and satiety cues, and adjust your food choices and portion sizes accordingly. Trust your body's signals and make choices that support your overall well-being.

15. Be Prepared for Challenges: Understand that following the Atkins diet may present challenges, especially in social situations or when dining out. Arm yourself

with strategies for navigating these challenges, such as choosing low-carb options, bringing your own food to events, or politely declining foods that don't align with your dietary goals.

16. Focus on Non-Scale Victories: While weight loss may be a primary goal of the Atkins diet, remember to celebrate non-scale victories as well. These could include improvements in energy levels, mood, sleep quality, physical fitness, or overall health markers such as blood sugar levels and cholesterol levels.

17. Emphasize Whole Health: Take a holistic approach to health and wellness by prioritizing factors beyond just diet and exercise. Focus on getting enough sleep, managing stress levels, nurturing social connections, and engaging in activities that bring you joy and fulfillment. A balanced approach to overall health can support your long-term success on the Atkins diet.

18. Reevaluate Goals Regularly: Regularly reassess your goals and motivations for following the Atkins diet. As your circumstances, preferences, and priorities evolve, your goals may also change. Be open to adjusting your approach to align with your current needs and aspirations.

19. Stay Consistent with Maintenance Phases: As you progress through the different phases of the Atkins diet, such as the ongoing weight loss (OWL) phase and the pre-maintenance and maintenance phases, stay consistent with your dietary choices and habits. These phases are designed to help you transition to a sustainable long-term eating pattern.

20. Practice Long-Term Thinking: Keep your long-term health and well-being in mind as you navigate your journey on the Atkins diet. Focus on building healthy habits that you can maintain for life rather than seeking quick fixes or short-term solutions. Remember that sustainable changes take time and patience.

Chapter 10: Sample Meal Plans and Recipes

<u>Breakfast, lunch, dinner, and snack ideas for each phase</u>

Here are sample meal plans and recipes tailored for an Atkins diet patient, focusing on low-carb, nutrient-dense foods:

 Sample Meal Plan 1: Induction Phase

Breakfast:

- Scrambled eggs cooked in butter with spinach and feta cheese
- Side of avocado slices

Lunch:

- Grilled chicken Caesar salad with romaine lettuce, grilled chicken breast, Parmesan cheese, and Caesar dressing (made with olive oil, anchovies, garlic, and lemon juice)
- Side of steamed broccoli

Dinner:

- Baked salmon with lemon and herbs
- Roasted asparagus with olive oil and garlic
- Mixed greens salad with cherry tomatoes, cucumber, and vinaigrette dressing

Snack:

- Celery sticks with almond butter

Sample Meal Plan 2: Ongoing Weight Loss (OWL) Phase

Breakfast:

- Greek yogurt with sliced strawberries and a sprinkle of chia seeds

- Low-carb protein shake made with almond milk, protein powder, and a handful of spinach

Lunch:

- Turkey and avocado lettuce wraps with turkey slices, avocado, lettuce, and mustard

- Side of cucumber slices with hummus

Dinner:

- Zucchini noodles (zoodles) with marinara sauce and grilled chicken breast

- Side of sautéed spinach with garlic and olive oil

Snack:

- Cottage cheese with sliced cucumber and cherry tomatoes

Sample Meal Plan 3: Pre-Maintenance/Maintenance Phase

Breakfast:

- Mushroom and spinach omelet cooked in coconut oil

- Side of mixed berries

Lunch:

- Cauliflower rice stir-fry with shrimp, mixed vegetables, and soy sauce

- Side of sliced bell peppers with guacamole

Dinner:

- Grilled steak with chimichurri sauce (made with fresh parsley, cilantro, garlic, olive oil, and vinegar)
- Roasted Brussels sprouts with bacon and balsamic glaze

Snack:

- Hard-boiled eggs with a sprinkle of sea salt

Low-Carb Recipes:

1. Zucchini Noodles with Pesto and Cherry Tomatoes:
   - Spiralize zucchini into noodles and sauté in olive oil until tender. Toss with homemade pesto (made with basil, garlic, pine nuts, Parmesan cheese, and olive oil) and halved cherry tomatoes.

2. Baked Chicken Parmesan:
   - Bread chicken breasts in a mixture of almond flour, Parmesan cheese, and Italian seasoning. Bake until golden and crispy. Top with marinara sauce and mozzarella cheese, and bake until bubbly.

3. Cauliflower Fried Rice:
   - Pulse cauliflower florets in a food processor until they resemble rice. Sauté with mixed vegetables, scrambled eggs, and soy sauce. Add cooked shrimp or chicken for extra protein.

4. Grilled Lemon Herb Salmon:

- Marinate salmon fillets in a mixture of lemon juice, olive oil, garlic, and fresh herbs (such as dill or parsley). Grill until cooked through and serve with a squeeze of fresh lemon.

5. Avocado Tuna Salad:

   - Mix canned tuna with diced avocado, celery, red onion, and mayonnaise. Season with salt, pepper, and lemon juice. Serve over a bed of mixed greens or in lettuce cups.

Sample Meal Plan 4: Pre-Maintenance/Maintenance Phase

Breakfast:
- Veggie and cheese omelet made with eggs, bell peppers, onions, and cheddar cheese
- Side of sliced avocado

Lunch:
- Grilled shrimp skewers with bell peppers and onions
- Side of Greek salad with cucumber, tomato, olives, feta cheese, and vinaigrette dressing

Dinner:
- Baked chicken thighs with rosemary and garlic
- Cauliflower mash with butter and Parmesan cheese
- Steamed green beans with almonds

Snack:

- Sugar-free Greek yogurt with a sprinkle of cinnamon and chopped nuts

Sample Meal Plan 5: Pre-Maintenance/Maintenance Phase

Breakfast:
- Low-carb breakfast burrito made with scrambled eggs, sautéed spinach, and crumbled bacon wrapped in a low-carb tortilla
- Side of salsa

Lunch:
- Turkey and avocado lettuce wraps with turkey slices, avocado, lettuce, and mayonnaise
- Side of cucumber slices with ranch dressing

Dinner:
- Grilled steak with garlic butter
- Roasted cauliflower with cumin and paprika
- Mixed greens salad with radishes, carrots, and blue cheese dressing

Snack:
- Celery sticks with cream cheese and smoked salmon

Low-Carb Recipes:

6. Eggplant Lasagna:

- Thinly slice eggplant lengthwise and grill until tender. Layer the eggplant slices with marinara sauce, ricotta cheese, mozzarella cheese, and Parmesan cheese. Bake until bubbly and golden.

7. Stuffed Bell Peppers:

   - Cut bell peppers in half and remove seeds. Fill with a mixture of cooked ground beef or turkey, cauliflower rice, diced tomatoes, onions, and spices. Top with shredded cheese and bake until peppers are tender.

8. Cauliflower Crust Pizza:

   - Make a low-carb pizza crust using cauliflower rice, eggs, Parmesan cheese, and Italian seasoning. Top with marinara sauce, cheese, and your favorite pizza toppings. Bake until cheese is melted and bubbly.

9. Lemon Garlic Butter Shrimp:

   - Sauté shrimp in butter with minced garlic, lemon juice, and parsley until cooked through. Serve with a side of steamed broccoli or asparagus.

10. Mediterranean Tuna Salad:

   - Mix canned tuna with diced cucumber, cherry tomatoes, red onion, Kalamata olives, feta cheese, olive oil, lemon juice, and oregano. Serve over a bed of mixed greens or in lettuce cups.

Here are alternative breakfast, lunch, dinner, and snack ideas for each phase of the Atkins diet:

Induction Phase (Phase 1):

Breakfast:

- Mushroom and spinach omelet cooked in coconut oil
- Side of sliced avocado

Lunch:

- Tuna salad lettuce wraps with canned tuna, mayonnaise, celery, and spices wrapped in lettuce leaves
- Side of cucumber slices with ranch dressing

Dinner:

- Baked chicken thighs with Cajun seasoning
- Steamed broccoli with garlic butter

Snack:

- Celery sticks with cream cheese and smoked salmon

Ongoing Weight Loss (OWL) Phase (Phase 2):

Breakfast:

- Greek yogurt with sliced strawberries and a sprinkle of chia seeds
- Low-carb protein smoothie made with almond milk, protein powder, and spinach

Lunch:

- Turkey and cheese roll-ups with sliced turkey, cheese, and mustard rolled up in lettuce leaves
- Side of cherry tomatoes with balsamic vinegar

Dinner:

- Grilled salmon with lemon and dill

- Roasted Brussels sprouts with bacon and Parmesan cheese

Snack:

- Hard-boiled eggs with a sprinkle of sea salt

Pre-Maintenance Phase (Phase 3):

Breakfast:

- Low-carb breakfast burrito made with scrambled eggs, sautéed bell peppers and onions, and crumbled sausage wrapped in a low-carb tortilla

- Side of salsa

Lunch:

- Chicken Caesar salad with grilled chicken breast, romaine lettuce, Parmesan cheese, and Caesar dressing (made with olive oil, anchovies, garlic, and lemon juice)

- Side of avocado slices

Dinner:

- Beef stir-fry with mixed vegetables and soy sauce

- Cauliflower rice with chopped scallions

Snack:

- Cottage cheese with sliced cucumber and cherry tomatoes

Maintenance Phase (Phase 4):

Breakfast:
- Veggie and cheese frittata made with eggs, bell peppers, onions, spinach, and cheddar cheese
- Side of mixed berries

Lunch:
- Shrimp and avocado salad with mixed greens, grilled shrimp, avocado slices, cherry tomatoes, and vinaigrette dressing
- Side of sliced almonds

Dinner:
- Grilled steak with chimichurri sauce (made with fresh parsley, cilantro, garlic, olive oil, and vinegar)
- Sautéed green beans with almonds

Snack:
- Sugar-free Greek yogurt with a sprinkle of cinnamon and chopped nuts

Certainly! Here are more breakfast, lunch, dinner, and snack ideas for each phase of the Atkins diet:

Induction Phase (Phase 1):

Breakfast:

- Smoked salmon and cream cheese roll-ups with cucumber slices

- Side of scrambled eggs cooked in butter

Lunch:

- Chicken and avocado salad with mixed greens, grilled chicken breast, avocado slices, and vinaigrette dressing

- Side of celery sticks with almond butter

Dinner:

- Baked cod with lemon and herbs

- Steamed asparagus with hollandaise sauce

Snack:

- Hard-boiled eggs with a sprinkle of salt and pepper

Ongoing Weight Loss (OWL) Phase (Phase 2):

Breakfast:

- Low-carb pancakes made with almond flour and served with sugar-free syrup

- Side of Greek yogurt with chopped nuts and a drizzle of honey

Lunch:

- Turkey and cheese lettuce wraps with turkey slices, cheese, lettuce, and mustard

- Side of cherry tomatoes with mozzarella cheese and basil

Dinner:

- Grilled chicken thighs with barbecue sauce

- Roasted cauliflower with Parmesan cheese and garlic

Snack:

- Celery sticks with cream cheese and sunflower seeds

Pre-Maintenance Phase (Phase 3):

Breakfast:

- Veggie and cheese scramble with eggs, bell peppers, onions, spinach, and feta cheese
- Side of sliced avocado

Lunch:

- Shrimp and broccoli stir-fry with garlic and ginger
- Side of mixed berries

Dinner:

- Beef and vegetable kabobs with bell peppers, onions, and mushrooms
- Cauliflower mash with butter and chives

Snack:

- Cottage cheese with sliced strawberries and a sprinkle of cinnamon

Maintenance Phase (Phase 4):

Breakfast:

- Spinach and mushroom frittata with eggs, spinach, mushrooms, and goat cheese

- Side of sliced tomatoes

Lunch:

- Salmon and avocado salad with mixed greens, grilled salmon, avocado slices, and lemon vinaigrette dressing
- Side of cucumber slices with hummus

Dinner:

- Grilled steak with garlic herb butter
- Sautéed spinach with pine nuts and raisins

Snack:

- Sugar-free yogurt with a handful of mixed nuts

<u>Delicious and easy-to-follow recipes</u>

Here are some delicious and easy-to-follow recipes suitable for an Atkins diet patient:

1. Grilled Lemon Herb Chicken:
  - Ingredients:
    - 4 boneless, skinless chicken breasts
    - 2 tablespoons olive oil
    - 2 cloves garlic, minced
    - 2 tablespoons chopped fresh herbs (such as rosemary, thyme, or parsley)
    - Juice of 1 lemon
    - Salt and pepper to taste
  - Instructions:

1. In a small bowl, mix together olive oil, minced garlic, chopped herbs, lemon juice, salt, and pepper.

2. Place chicken breasts in a shallow dish and pour the marinade over them, turning to coat evenly. Cover and refrigerate for at least 30 minutes.

3. Preheat grill to medium-high heat. Grill chicken breasts for 6-8 minutes per side, or until cooked through and no longer pink in the center.

4. Serve grilled chicken breasts with your favorite low-carb side dishes, such as roasted vegetables or cauliflower rice.

2. Zucchini Noodles with Pesto and Cherry Tomatoes:
   - Ingredients:
     - 4 medium zucchini, spiralized into noodles
     - 1 cup cherry tomatoes, halved
     - 1/4 cup homemade or store-bought pesto sauce
     - 2 tablespoons grated Parmesan cheese
     - Salt and pepper to taste
   - Instructions:

1. In a large skillet, heat olive oil over medium heat. Add spiralized zucchini noodles and cook for 2-3 minutes, or until just tender.

2. Add cherry tomatoes to the skillet and cook for an additional 1-2 minutes, until heated through.

3. Remove skillet from heat and stir in pesto sauce until well combined.

4. Divide zucchini noodles and cherry tomatoes among serving plates. Sprinkle with grated Parmesan cheese and season with salt and pepper to taste.

3. Baked Salmon with Dill and Lemon:
   - Ingredients:

- 4 salmon fillets

- 2 tablespoons olive oil

- 2 cloves garlic, minced

- 2 tablespoons chopped fresh dill

- Juice of 1 lemon

- Salt and pepper to taste

- Instructions:

1. Preheat oven to 375°F (190°C). Line a baking sheet with parchment paper.

2. Place salmon fillets on the prepared baking sheet. Drizzle with olive oil and sprinkle minced garlic, chopped dill, and lemon juice over the top.

3. Season salmon fillets with salt and pepper to taste.

4. Bake in preheated oven for 12-15 minutes, or until salmon is cooked through and flakes easily with a fork.

5. Serve baked salmon with your favorite low-carb side dishes, such as steamed vegetables or a green salad.

4. Low-Carb Cauliflower Fried Rice:

- Ingredients:

- 1 medium head cauliflower, grated into rice-like grains

- 2 tablespoons sesame oil

- 2 cloves garlic, minced

- 1 cup mixed vegetables (such as peas, carrots, and bell peppers)

- 2 eggs, lightly beaten

- 2 tablespoons soy sauce or tamari

- 2 green onions, thinly sliced

- Salt and pepper to taste

- Instructions:

1. In a large skillet or wok, heat sesame oil over medium heat. Add minced garlic and sauté for 1-2 minutes, until fragrant.

2. Add grated cauliflower and mixed vegetables to the skillet. Cook for 5-7 minutes, stirring occasionally, until vegetables are tender.

3. Push cauliflower mixture to one side of the skillet and pour beaten eggs into the empty side. Scramble eggs until cooked through, then mix with cauliflower mixture.

4. Stir in soy sauce or tamari and sliced green onions. Season with salt and pepper to taste.

5. Serve low-carb cauliflower fried rice as a main dish or as a side dish with your favorite protein.

5. Avocado and Bacon Egg Cups:

  - Ingredients:

    - 2 avocados, halved and pitted

    - 4 large eggs

    - 4 slices bacon, cooked and crumbled

    - Salt and pepper to taste

    - Fresh chives for garnish

  - Instructions:

    1. Preheat the oven to 375°F (190°C).

    2. Scoop out a small portion of each avocado half to create a well for the egg.

    3. Crack one egg into each avocado half. Season with salt and pepper.

    4. Place the avocado halves on a baking sheet and bake for 12-15 minutes or until the eggs are cooked to your liking.

    5. Sprinkle crumbled bacon on top, garnish with fresh chives, and serve.

6. Cauliflower and Broccoli Cheese Casserole:

   - Ingredients:

     - 2 cups cauliflower florets

     - 2 cups broccoli florets

     - 1 cup shredded cheddar cheese

     - 1/2 cup heavy cream

     - 2 tablespoons cream cheese

     - 1 teaspoon Dijon mustard

     - Salt and pepper to taste

   - Instructions:

     1. Preheat the oven to 375°F (190°C).

     2. Steam cauliflower and broccoli until tender.

     3. In a saucepan over medium heat, combine heavy cream, cream cheese, and Dijon mustard. Stir until smooth.

     4. Place steamed cauliflower and broccoli in a baking dish, pour the cheese sauce over them, and mix well.

     5. Sprinkle shredded cheddar cheese on top and bake for 20-25 minutes or until bubbly and golden.

7. Turkey and Avocado Lettuce Wraps:

   - Ingredients:

     - 1 pound ground turkey

     - 1 tablespoon olive oil

     - 1 teaspoon taco seasoning

     - Iceberg lettuce leaves

     - 1 avocado, sliced

     - Salsa for topping

- Instructions:

   1. In a skillet over medium heat, cook ground turkey in olive oil until browned. Season with taco seasoning.

   2. Spoon the turkey mixture onto iceberg lettuce leaves.

   3. Top each lettuce wrap with sliced avocado and salsa.

8. Eggplant Lasagna:

  - Ingredients:

    - 1 large eggplant, sliced thinly

    - 1 pound ground beef

    - 1 cup marinara sauce

    - 1 cup ricotta cheese

    - 1 cup shredded mozzarella cheese

    - 1/4 cup grated Parmesan cheese

    - Fresh basil for garnish

  - Instructions:

   1. Preheat the oven to 375°F (190°C).

   2. Grill or bake eggplant slices until tender.

   3. In a skillet, cook ground beef until browned. Stir in marinara sauce.

   4. In a baking dish, layer eggplant slices, ground beef mixture, ricotta cheese, and mozzarella cheese. Repeat until all ingredients are used.

   5. Top with grated Parmesan cheese and bake for 25-30 minutes or until bubbly and golden. Garnish with fresh basil before serving.

9. Cajun Shrimp and Cauliflower Rice:

  - Ingredients:

    - 1 pound shrimp, peeled and deveined

- 2 tablespoons Cajun seasoning

- 1 tablespoon olive oil

- 4 cups cauliflower rice

- 1 bell pepper, diced

- 1/2 cup diced tomatoes

- Fresh parsley for garnish

- Instructions:

1. In a bowl, toss shrimp with Cajun seasoning.

2. Heat olive oil in a skillet over medium-high heat. Add shrimp and cook until pink and opaque.

3. In the same skillet, add cauliflower rice, bell pepper, and diced tomatoes. Cook until vegetables are tender.

4. Serve Cajun shrimp over cauliflower rice and garnish with fresh parsley.

10. Creamy Spinach and Artichoke Chicken:

  - Ingredients:

    - 4 boneless, skinless chicken breasts

    - 1 cup creamed spinach and artichoke dip

    - 1/2 cup shredded mozzarella cheese

    - 1/4 cup grated Parmesan cheese

    - Salt and pepper to taste

  - Instructions:

  1. Preheat the oven to 375°F (190°C).

  2. Season chicken breasts with salt and pepper and place them in a baking dish.

  3. Spread creamed spinach and artichoke dip over the chicken breasts.

  4. Sprinkle shredded mozzarella and grated Parmesan cheese on top.

5. Bake for 25-30 minutes or until the chicken is cooked through and the cheese is bubbly and golden.

<u>Nutritional information for each recipe</u>

Here's the nutritional information for each recipe mentioned earlier, tailored for an Atkins diet patient. Please note that these values are approximate and may vary based on specific ingredients and portion sizes:

1. Grilled Lemon Herb Chicken:
   - Per serving (1 chicken breast):
     - Calories: 250
     - Protein: 30g
     - Fat: 12g
     - Carbohydrates: 1g
     - Fiber: 0g
     - Net Carbs: 1g

2. Zucchini Noodles with Pesto and Cherry Tomatoes:
   - Per serving (1/4 of the recipe):
     - Calories: 150
     - Protein: 3g
     - Fat: 12g
     - Carbohydrates: 8g
     - Fiber: 3g
     - Net Carbs: 5g

3. Baked Salmon with Dill and Lemon:

- Per serving (1 fillet):

  - Calories: 300

  - Protein: 25g

  - Fat: 20g

  - Carbohydrates: 1g

  - Fiber: 0g

  - Net Carbs: 1g

4. Low-Carb Cauliflower Fried Rice:

  - Per serving (1/4 of the recipe):

    - Calories: 150

    - Protein: 5g

    - Fat: 9g

    - Carbohydrates: 10g

    - Fiber: 4g

    - Net Carbs: 6g

5. Avocado and Bacon Egg Cups:

  - Per serving (1 egg cup):

    - Calories: 180

    - Protein: 8g

    - Fat: 15g

    - Carbohydrates: 4g

    - Fiber: 3g

    - Net Carbs: 1g

6. Cauliflower and Broccoli Cheese Casserole:

- Per serving (1/4 of the casserole):

  - Calories: 200

  - Protein: 10g

  - Fat: 15g

  - Carbohydrates: 7g

  - Fiber: 3g

  - Net Carbs: 4g

7. Turkey and Avocado Lettuce Wraps:

  - Per serving (2 lettuce wraps):

  - Calories: 250

  - Protein: 20g

  - Fat: 15g

  - Carbohydrates: 6g

  - Fiber: 4g

  - Net Carbs: 2g

8. Eggplant Lasagna:

  - Per serving (1/4 of the lasagna):

  - Calories: 300

  - Protein: 18g

  - Fat: 20g

  - Carbohydrates: 12g

  - Fiber: 5g

  - Net Carbs: 7g

9. Cajun Shrimp and Cauliflower Rice:

- Per serving (1/4 of the recipe):

  - Calories: 200

  - Protein: 15g

  - Fat: 10g

  - Carbohydrates: 9g

  - Fiber: 4g

  - Net Carbs: 5g

10. Creamy Spinach and Artichoke Chicken:

  - Per serving (1 chicken breast):

    - Calories: 350

    - Protein: 30g

    - Fat: 20g

    - Carbohydrates: 8g

    - Fiber: 3g

    - Net Carbs: 5g

11. Grilled Lemon Herb Chicken:

  - Per serving (1 chicken breast):

    - Calories: 250

    - Protein: 30g

    - Fat: 12g

    - Carbohydrates: 1g

    - Fiber: 0g

    - Net Carbs: 1g

12. Zucchini Noodles with Pesto and Cherry Tomatoes:

- Per serving (1/4 of the recipe):

    - Calories: 150

    - Protein: 3g

    - Fat: 12g

    - Carbohydrates: 8g

    - Fiber: 3g

    - Net Carbs: 5g

13. Baked Salmon with Dill and Lemon:

  - Per serving (1 fillet):

    - Calories: 300

    - Protein: 25g

    - Fat: 20g

    - Carbohydrates: 1g

    - Fiber: 0g

    - Net Carbs: 1g

14. Low-Carb Cauliflower Fried Rice:

  - Per serving (1/4 of the recipe):

    - Calories: 150

    - Protein: 5g

    - Fat: 9g

    - Carbohydrates: 10g

    - Fiber: 4g

    - Net Carbs: 6g

15. Avocado and Bacon Egg Cups:

- Per serving (1 egg cup):

  - Calories: 180

  - Protein: 8g

  - Fat: 15g

  - Carbohydrates: 4g

  - Fiber: 3g

  - Net Carbs: 1g

16. Cauliflower and Broccoli Cheese Casserole:

  - Per serving (1/4 of the casserole):

    - Calories: 200

    - Protein: 10g

    - Fat: 15g

    - Carbohydrates: 7g

    - Fiber: 3g

    - Net Carbs: 4g

17. Turkey and Avocado Lettuce Wraps:

  - Per serving (2 lettuce wraps):

    - Calories: 250

    - Protein: 20g

    - Fat: 15g

    - Carbohydrates: 6g

    - Fiber: 4g

    - Net Carbs: 2g

18. Eggplant Lasagna:

- Per serving (1/4 of the lasagna):

  - Calories: 300

  - Protein: 18g

  - Fat: 20g

  - Carbohydrates: 12g

  - Fiber: 5g

  - Net Carbs: 7g

19. Cajun Shrimp and Cauliflower Rice:

  - Per serving (1/4 of the recipe):

  - Calories: 200

  - Protein: 15g

  - Fat: 10g

  - Carbohydrates: 9g

  - Fiber: 4g

  - Net Carbs: 5g

20. Creamy Spinach and Artichoke Chicken:

  - Per serving (1 chicken breast):

  - Calories: 350

  - Protein: 30g

  - Fat: 20g

  - Carbohydrates: 8g

  - Fiber: 3g

  - Net Carbs: 5g

These nutritional values are calculated per serving and are based on standard portions.

Chapter 11: Conclusion

Reflecting on your Atkins journey

Reflecting on your Atkins journey can be a valuable practice to understand your progress, challenges, and successes throughout the process. Here are some steps you can take to reflect on your Atkins journey:

1. Set aside time: Find a quiet and comfortable space where you can reflect without distractions. Set aside dedicated time to focus on your thoughts and experiences.

2. Review your goals: Start by revisiting the goals you set at the beginning of your Atkins journey. Consider why you embarked on this dietary approach, whether it was for weight loss, improved health, or other reasons.

3. Assess your progress: Reflect on how far you've come since starting the Atkins diet. Consider any changes in your weight, energy levels, mood, and overall well-being. Take note of both physical and non-physical changes you've observed.

4. Identify challenges: Reflect on any obstacles or challenges you encountered along the way. This could include cravings, social situations, dining out, or adjusting to new eating habits. Consider how you overcame these challenges and what strategies were effective.

5. Celebrate successes: Acknowledge and celebrate your successes, no matter how small they may seem. This could be reaching a weight loss milestone, sticking to your meal plan during a challenging week, or making healthier food choices.

6. Learn from setbacks: Reflect on any setbacks or slip-ups you experienced during your Atkins journey. Instead of dwelling on them, use them as learning opportunities. Consider what triggered the setback and how you can prevent similar situations in the future.

7. Evaluate your satisfaction: Reflect on your overall satisfaction with the Atkins diet. Consider whether you enjoy the foods you're eating, how sustainable the diet feels for you, and whether you're experiencing any negative side effects.

8. Consider adjustments: Based on your reflections, consider whether any adjustments are needed to optimize your Atkins journey. This could include tweaking your meal plan, seeking additional support or resources, or incorporating more physical activity.

9. Set new goals: Based on your reflections, set new goals for your Atkins journey moving forward. These could be related to weight loss, improved health markers, increased physical activity, or other aspects of your well-being.

10. Practice self-compassion: Remember to be kind to yourself throughout this process. Celebrate your successes, learn from your challenges, and embrace the journey with self-compassion and positivity.

Reflecting on your Atkins journey involves more than just assessing your physical progress. It also entails examining the mental, emotional, and social aspects of your experience. Here are some additional points to consider when reflecting on your Atkins journey:

1. Mindful Eating: Reflect on how your relationship with food has evolved since starting the Atkins diet. Have you become more mindful of your eating habits, such as paying attention to hunger and fullness cues? How has your awareness of food choices impacted your overall well-being?

2. Emotional Well-being: Consider how the Atkins diet has influenced your emotional well-being. Have you noticed any changes in your mood, stress levels, or emotional resilience? Reflect on whether the dietary changes have had a positive or negative impact on your mental health.

3. Social Dynamics: Reflect on how your social interactions and relationships have been affected by the Atkins diet. Have you faced any challenges or judgments from friends, family, or colleagues regarding your dietary choices? How have you navigated social situations, such as dining out or attending social gatherings, while following the Atkins diet?

4. Self-Discovery: Take time to reflect on what you've learned about yourself throughout your Atkins journey. Have you discovered new strengths, habits, or preferences related to your health and well-being? How have you adapted to changes in your lifestyle and dietary habits?

5. Long-Term Sustainability: Consider the long-term sustainability of the Atkins diet for your lifestyle and goals. Reflect on whether the dietary principles align with your values and preferences for long-term health and well-being. Are there any adjustments or modifications you need to make to ensure the sustainability of your dietary approach?

6. Gratitude: Express gratitude for the progress you've made and the support you've received along your Atkins journey. Reflect on the positive aspects of your experience, such as improved health markers, increased energy levels, or enhanced self-confidence. Acknowledge the efforts you've invested in prioritizing your health and well-being.

7. Continued Growth: Embrace your Atkins journey as an ongoing process of growth and self-discovery. Reflect on how you can continue to evolve and improve your health habits moving forward. Set new goals, explore new recipes and foods, and remain open to learning and adapting as you navigate your health journey.

<u>Final words of encouragement and advice</u>

As you continue your Atkins journey, remember that you are making positive changes for your health and well-being. Here are some final words of encouragement and advice to support you along the way:

1. Stay Consistent: Consistency is key to success on the Atkins diet. Stick to your meal plan, make mindful food choices, and stay committed to your health goals. Remember that small, consistent efforts can lead to significant results over time.

2. Listen to Your Body: Pay attention to your body's signals of hunger, fullness, and satisfaction. Eat when you're hungry, stop when you're full, and choose foods that nourish your body and make you feel your best. Trust your instincts and tune into your body's needs.

3. Stay Positive: Maintain a positive mindset and focus on your progress, no matter how small. Celebrate your successes, learn from setbacks, and embrace the journey

with optimism and resilience. Surround yourself with positivity and support to stay motivated and inspired.

4. Be Patient: Remember that meaningful changes take time. Trust the process and be patient with yourself as you navigate your Atkins journey. Results may not happen overnight, but with dedication and perseverance, you will reach your goals.

5. Practice Self-Care: Prioritize self-care to support your overall well-being. Get plenty of rest, manage stress effectively, and engage in activities that bring you joy and relaxation. Taking care of yourself holistically will enhance your success on the Atkins diet.

6. Seek Support: Reach out to friends, family, or support groups for encouragement and accountability. Share your journey with others who understand and can offer guidance, motivation, and camaraderie along the way. Remember, you're not alone in this journey.

7. Stay Educated: Continue to educate yourself about the Atkins diet and healthy living. Stay informed about nutrition, new recipes, and lifestyle tips that align with your dietary approach. Knowledge is power, and staying educated will empower you to make informed choices for your health.

8. Celebrate Your Achievements: Take time to acknowledge and celebrate your achievements, no matter how small. Whether it's reaching a weight loss milestone, achieving better health markers, or mastering a new recipe, celebrate your progress and be proud of your accomplishments.

9. Stay Flexible: Be open to adjusting your approach as needed based on your individual needs and experiences. Your Atkins journey is unique to you, and it's important to adapt your plan to suit your lifestyle, preferences, and goals.

10. Believe in Yourself: Finally, believe in yourself and your ability to succeed. You have the strength, determination, and resilience to overcome challenges and achieve your health goals. Trust in yourself and your journey, and know that you are capable of creating the healthy and vibrant life you deserve.

11. Embrace Variety: Explore a wide range of low-carb foods and recipes to keep your meals interesting and satisfying. Don't be afraid to experiment with new ingredients and flavors to spice up your meals and prevent boredom.

12. Stay Hydrated: Remember to drink plenty of water throughout the day to stay hydrated and support your body's functions. Hydration is important for overall health and can help with weight management and appetite control.

13. Be Mindful of Portions: Pay attention to portion sizes to ensure you're not overeating, even when enjoying low-carb foods. Practice mindful eating by listening to your body's hunger and fullness cues to avoid overindulging.

14. Plan Ahead: Take time to plan your meals and snacks in advance to avoid impulse eating and make healthier choices. Stock your kitchen with Atkins-friendly foods and snacks to stay on track even when you're busy or on the go.

15. Focus on Non-Scale Victories: While weight loss may be a primary goal, remember to celebrate non-scale victories as well. Notice improvements in energy levels, mood, sleep quality, and overall well-being as indicators of your progress.

16. Stay Active: Incorporate regular physical activity into your routine to complement your Atkins diet and support your overall health. Find activities you enjoy, such as walking, cycling, or strength training, and make movement a priority in your daily life.

17. Practice Patience: Be patient with yourself and your body as you progress on your Atkins journey. Weight loss and health improvements take time, and it's important to trust the process and stay committed to your goals.

18. Celebrate Milestones: Set small, achievable milestones along your journey and celebrate each one as you reach them. Whether it's losing a certain amount of weight, fitting into a smaller clothing size, or achieving a health goal, acknowledge your achievements and reward yourself for your hard work.

19. Stay Inspired: Surround yourself with inspiration and motivation to stay on track with your Atkins journey. Follow social media accounts, join online communities, and read success stories to stay inspired and motivated to reach your goals.

20. Be Kind to Yourself: Finally, remember to be kind to yourself throughout your Atkins journey. Treat yourself with compassion and understanding, and don't be too hard on yourself if you encounter setbacks or challenges. Every step forward is progress, and you're doing the best you can for your health and well-being.

www.ingramcontent.com/pod-product-compliance
Lightning Source LLC
Chambersburg PA
CBHW080718260726
48660CB00010B/3596